Decon-structing the Fitness Industrial Complex

HOW TO RESIST, DISRUPT, AND

RECLAIM WHAT IT MEANS TO

BE FIT IN AMERICAN CULTURE

Edited by Justice Roe Williams,
Roc Rochon, and Lawrence Koval

North Atlantic Books
Huichin, unceded Ohlone land
aka Berkeley, California

Published by
North Atlantic Books
Huichin, unceded Ohlone land
aka Berkeley, California

Cover art and design by Amanda Weiss
Book design by Happenstance-Type-O-Rama

Printed in Canada

Deconstructing the Fitness-Industrial Complex: How to Resist, Disrupt, and Reclaim What It Means to Be Fit in American Culture is sponsored and published by North Atlantic Books, an educational nonprofit based in the unceded Ohlone land Huichin (*aka* Berkeley, CA) that collaborates with partners to develop cross-cultural perspectives; nurture holistic views of art, science, the humanities, and healing; and seed personal and global transformation by publishing work on the relationship of body, spirit, and nature.

North Atlantic Books' publications are distributed to the US trade and internationally by Penguin Random House Publisher Services. For further information, visit our website at www.northatlanticbooks.com.

Library of Congress Cataloging-in-Publication Data

Names: Rochon, Roc, editor. | Koval, Lawrence, editor. | Williams, Justice, editor.
Title: Deconstructing the fitness-industrial complex : how to resist, disrupt, and reclaim what it means to be fit in American culture / Justice Williams, Roc Rochon, and Lawrence Koval.
Description: Berkeley, CA : North Atlantic Books, [2023] | Includes bibliographical references and index.
Identifiers: LCCN 2022047926 (print) | LCCN 2022047927 (ebook) | ISBN 9781623177270 (trade paperback) | ISBN 9781623177287 (ebook)
Subjects: LCSH: Physical fitness—Social aspects—United States. | Physical fitness—Psychological aspects—United States. | Physical fitness centers—United States. | Social integration—United States. | Minorities—United States—Social conditions. | Sexual minorities—United States—Social conditions.
Classification: LCC GV342.27 .D43 2023 (print) | LCC GV342.27 (ebook) | DDC 306.4/613—dc23/eng/20221103
LC record available at https://lccn.loc.gov/2022047926
LC ebook record available at https://lccn.loc.gov/2022047927

1 2 3 4 5 6 7 8 9 MARQUIS 27 26 25 24 23

North Atlantic Books is committed to the protection of our environment. We print on recycled paper whenever possible and partner with printers who strive to use environmentally responsible practices.

Contents

PART III

How We Empowered Ourselves to Move Forward and Help Our Communities Polish Their Armor   101

Acknowledgments

JUSTICE ROE WILLIAMS

I want to first thank my mother for showering me with unconditional love and modeling what that love looks like across relationships. She is my Rock! I also want to acknowledge that the land we call the United States of America is the ancestral territory of the Indigenous Nations, who are the continuous stewards of this land. I pay respect to their ancestors and descendants. I recognize that this land remains scarred by a history of colonial violence and displacement, yet in spite of all this, Indigenous Nations have remained deeply connected to this land. I recognize that I am a "guest" and it's my responsibility to continue to learn about, support, and amplify Indigenous voices and cultural work in all the ways that I can.

As a coach, one of the first things I realized is that I wear several different hats during each training session. Sometimes coaching sessions become impromptu therapy. I am so grateful for my clients, colleagues, and friends who allowed me to be a part of their fitness journeys. This book is dedicated to them. We grew as a moving community, and they helped me shift my views and ideals of what it means to create inclusive gym spaces.

I am so humbled to have had the opportunity to work with my co-editors on this book. This project is the culmination of eight years of hard work and dedication. In that time I have been in community with some really phenomenal individuals who helped me to create this anthology. Roc has been much like a rock for me over the course of this project. I am so honored to know someone with such genius—such a phenomenal thinker. I am fortunate to have them as a co-editor. They have served as a mirror especially for the times that I needed reflection. I have watched them grow and cultivate powerful communities and movement spaces as the founder of Rooted Resistance. In our long journey as friends, we have collectively been shifting the narrative of what it means to move, honor, and celebrate our bodies.

I am very lucky to have met Lawrence when I did. When we met, I was just beginning my work with Fitness 4 All Bodies. Lawrence supported me in this vision and helped me even when my ideas seemed beyond reach. When I look back to 2020, when this work was community workouts for the Queer Gym Pop Up and panel discussions, now, two years later this has grown to a number of courses including our six-week course and finally this anthology. I am grateful and humbled to be in community with Lawrence, who has taught me so much about myself in this work. There is something about working with amazing people: you get to do some truly amazing things. This project would not be without him.

Over the past two years I have had the distinct opportunity to meet some really amazing coaches, trainers, and activists within the field who are now the authors in this book. I am so honored to be connected to each of them. Throughout the course of the year, I have had the opportunity of taking courses from some, facilitating courses with others, and a few of them were a part of our panel discussions about creating inclusive fitness spaces. I even had the opportunity to join a movement course with some, and it was the very model of what I would want to see in all movement spaces.

Some of these coaches, trainers, and activists are contributors to this text. An anthology like this cannot be made without an incredible group of writers who are dedicated to this work. I want to thank them all for their willingness to not just write their pieces and the time that takes, but to share their stories and experiences, many of which are vulnerable and personal.

I want to thank Ilya Parker, Chrissy King, Shannon Wagner, the Women's Strength Coalition, Jack Juris, Jason and Lauren Pak for their ongoing activism within the field and their support of the work and vision of Fitness4AllBodies. Their inspiring examples remind me that we are a larger community with a shared vision to change fitness, making space for all bodies.

I also would like to take a moment to thank my Freeing Ourselves family: Jen Debarros, Cedric Josey, Stan Dominic, and Walter Grant and the New

Bedford Collective along with the Body Image 4 Justice collective: Nic McCaskill, Shawn Von Stowers, Mark Williams, and Chris Miller.

Thanks so much to Jo Quest-Neubert, Josh Gambrell, Mark Williams, Michelle Farrell, and Rosevan for taking the time to read, make some edits, and give me some direction. This book definitely would not have happened without the love and care of my community.

I want to thank Dr. Joy Cox for being there for me every time I called. When we met, we became fast friends. She has been a godsend to the community, and I have been honored to work with her on a couple of community projects throughout the year. It is in many ways because of Joy that I was blessed with this opportunity.

And I can't forget to thank my mom, who is always on my side and has shown me what love looks like!!!!

ROC ROCHON

To begin I am going to acknowledge physicality. I am located on unceded land that is the ancestral and traditional territory of the Apalachee Nation, the Muscogee Creek Nation, the Miccosukee Tribe of Florida, the Seminole Nation of Oklahoma, and the Seminole Tribe of Florida. The ongoing sociohistorical structure of settler colonial violence is embedded in the institutional practices in North America*. I recognize the ongoing relationships of care that Indigenous Nations maintain with this land and extend my gratitude. I recognize Black Natives who celebrate their Blackness and Indigeneity in wholeness. I recognize enslaved Africans and my ancestors who were kidnapped and held hostage from their homelands, brutalized, tortured, raped, and forced to labor on this land, in essence being confined and detained on this land.

I wrestle with what then becomes home for generations of descendants born, raised, and expected to live and flourish while encountering this memorial site of geographical bodily terror. I cannot admire the beauty of this land without simultaneously struggling with the vile colonial history this land

---

* Chen Chen and Daniel S. Mason, "Making Settler Colonialism Visible in Sport Management." *Journal of Sport Management* 33, no. 5 (September 2019): 379-392.

and the people of African descent on it have survived. In her "Touching the Earth" essay, bell hooks wrote, "When the Earth is sacred to us, our bodies can also be sacred to us." I believe in what my ancestors both human and nonhuman know to be true—that healing the body is inextricably connected to the healing of Earth. So to take seriously the project of "deconstructing fitness" means that we have to understand histories of Euro-American imperialism and the ways land, bodies, and cultures are weaponized against each other—deemed either superior or inferior. For whom and what is this dichotomy in service? And how has the fitness industry been complicit?

I want to graciously thank all the contributors to this book, each of whom offer the layered complexities to this question. Though several of us have met virtually, many of us have only been a part of email threads over the course of this project. I am in deep gratitude for the personal narratives that you all have willingly invited us to think, feel, and act in collaboration with. The writing process and recalling memories can sometimes be a place of tension, rage, joy, comfort, and even pain—thank you for your presence and holding all the emotions that may have come up for you throughout this project. To North Atlantic Books, thank you for the enthusiasm and support throughout each phase of the project.

Thank you to the co-editors of this book. It has been a privilege to think alongside you both throughout this project and beyond. Justice, I am so proud of you. Thank you for inviting me in to be a part of this project. Thank you for valuing the teaching and learning that I contribute within Critical Sport Studies. Your carework is something that I have seen lived out within the community from our Body Image 4 Justice Boston and western Massachusetts days—meeting you a decade ago contributed to my sense of self in adulthood and certainly to the inception of Rooted Resistance. Lawrence, what a journey this has been. I am grateful to have met you over the last few years and built a meaningful relationship. Thank you for the chance to support and witness you throughout your thesis work. Collaborating with you on this project has felt abundant. Thank you for your solidarity in and through the ongoing struggles of academia. May your creative imagination continue developing critical stories around the ways bodies are depicted in sport anime.

To Nicholas Hue McCaskill, Shawn Von Stowers, Ilya Parker, and Noori Jerrard, thank you. To all the Black queer, trans, and nonbinary people who assert their wholeness by allowing their bodies to take up space, be visible on their own terms, and in the process demonstrate that self-determination is an embodied practice.

To my parents and twin sibling who supported and encouraged play in my youth and even still in adult life. From sliding down the apartment complex hill in the snow, to neighborhood pick-up basketball games, to riding our bicycles, to local town recreation leagues, to collegiate and community-based movement and physical activity experiences—I cherish these moments and recognize the privilege I've had to access them. Thank you for reminding me early on what it means to stay rooted—you have taught me the possibilities of feeling liberation in and through my body.

LAWRENCE KOVAL

I want to humbly acknowledge that the land I live, work, and write this from is unceded land of Indigenous nations and peoples. For centuries, nations and their elders have served as stewards to this land only to be met with a multitude of violence that persists today. As Indigenous peoples have stated continuously, decolonization is not a metaphor, but an action that needs to be taken now to return Indigenous nations and peoples to their status as stewards of this land and to be able to live both safely and prosperously upon it.

I want to sincerely thank all the contributors in this book. For some, this was our first time meeting and working together, and for others, this was a continuation and development of our relationship. Either way, I am grateful to have an opportunity to work on a project of this nature—that is really the first of its kind—and to have been part of getting these essays prepared for publication, especially given how personal, rich, and vulnerable many of these pieces are. It makes me feel incredibly lucky and grateful to get to work closely with so many incredible activists, community members, and dreamers and to get their work out to more people.

I am grateful for the larger community of activists, leaders, and stewards within this industry who are committed to creating spaces and practices that disrupt the status quo and open up new possibilities of how we can connect and move together with each other, our bodies, and ourselves.

Out of this community, Justice and Roc are truly some of the greatest luminaries that I have had the privilege of working with. I am so grateful to have met you when I did, Justice! Much more, that our relationship has been able to grow into one defined by collaboration, community, and possibilities. You have taught me so much in the process and connected me to a world of incredible, loving, and supportive people. I am thrilled to see this anthology reach completion and for it to lift up your work that you have been dedicated to for so long!

Roc, you are my comrade in navigating all the bullshit that is academia and traversing the wildness that constitutes life! I am so grateful to have been able to work on this project alongside you. Every time I hear the way you are digesting information and the work that you are creating, I am struck by what a visionary you are. I am looking forward to this anthology being just the beginning of a long list of creations that come from your work in all forms! You have a kind, wise heart that is reflected in everything you do, and I am truly humbled to bear witness to it.

Introduction

ROC ROCHON

Through the narratives of activists, movement practitioners, therapists, fitness coaches, and trainers, *Deconstructing the Fitness-Industrial Complex: How to Resist, Disrupt, and Reclaim What It Means to Be Fit in American Culture* is a reclamation of our stories and the body. Each contribution to this anthology offers in-depth insights of lived experiences in relation to the sociohistorical context of the fitness industry. As you journey through the pages of this book, you will understand more about the practice of deconstructing the harm of the current fitness industry, as well as the liberatory practices that are shifting the future of fitness and health. For all of those who have been disembodied, erased, unseen, and who live/lived liminal experiences within the current fitness culture, we hope that through this storytelling you recognize the imperative of future possibilities.

A Brief History of the Movement

When the Body Image 4 Justice (BI4J) initiative, founded by Justice Roe Williams, began in August 2013, our focus was creating a revolutionary wellness center that met the needs of our diverse trans bodies, including creating access for trans individuals to be their authentic selves without abusing their bodies to do so. For us this meant creating access for trans individuals to receive bodywork and healthcare access, such as massage, personal training, hormone replacement therapy (HRT), medical transition prep, and knowledge about gender-affirming healthcare options in the greater Boston area.

BI4J had recognized that the resources available were neither culturally relevant nor meeting the needs of Black, Indigenous, Latiné/x, Asian, and other racialized groups of people. We created our own lane by reimagining spaces for cross-cultural and social justice dialogue. We were interested in engaging and amplifying the leadership of Black people and racialized people by making a space for trans bodies to feel safe and respected by working with bodywork practitioners. Our belief was, and still is, that if we meet the needs of Black transgender people and other racialized people, we will carve pathways to better meet the needs of all systemically oppressed groups who need access to healthcare.

In 2014 the first phase of this program was focused in the greater Boston area, facilitating workshops at the Black Trans Advocacy Conference and the Philadelphia Health Conference. Through building partnerships across the country, we were able to organize our first LGBTQAI+* Health and Wellness conference weekend, where we brought in massage, reiki, educational nutrition access, and personal trainers. This core group created focus groups to determine our long-term goal and vision, to bring forth a wellness center with a gym attachment. The focus groups captured several aspects regarding trans health, including gym use, locker room use, shower use, backroom use, access to massage, acupuncture, HRT, preparing for surgery, coping with binders and packers, navigating medical industry, and insurance coverage policies.

The second phase of the BI4J initiative was a fundraising campaign to create a temporary space for transgender individuals to have a safe environment to become physically active through both one-on-one and group training opportunities. This space would be open to all LGBTQAI+ people who were seeking a safe and restorative community space in Boston. The grand opening was in October 2015.

By organizing on the ground in Boston and spreading this work at national conferences, new BI4J chapters launched in New York, Georgia, North

---

* The LGBTQAI+ acronym stands for lesbian, gay, bisexual, transgender, queer, asexual or aromantic, and intersex. The + recognizes those whose sexualities expand beyond the acronym.

Carolina, Florida, and Texas to expand our vision nationwide. At the time we were developing a curriculum as a training guide for gym staff, fitness coaches, massage therapists, acupuncturists, and more. Our programming model for implementation had four essential components:

- Active health and fitness

- Mental health and wellness

- Curriculum development and training for trainers, bodyworkers, and practitioners

- Sharing knowledge and networking through local and national conferences

My comrade Justice Roe Williams frequently reflects on the ways in which we value Black trans and nonbinary experiences collectively. When sharing about his life, he often begins from drawing upon his experiences being introduced to the Four I's of Oppression and the 10 C's Model at Springfield College in Massachusetts and their application in his life.[1] Elaborating on this framework has become a guide for his approach to inclusive fitness. Justice uses the 10 C's to help facilitate the discussion of learning about ourselves and validating our own lives. The 10 C's represent five areas of awareness: color, culture, class, character, and context. The remaining five areas represent avenues to create and sustain change: confidence, courage, commitment, conflict, and community. A key component to Justice's application of the Four I's framework is to understand the ways that we have learned about ourselves, our bodies, and the ways we are in relationship with others in our local community and in the world. These two frameworks inspire Justice's practices and the ways he thinks about social change. He places emphasis on understanding that these systems are undoubtably intertwined and are often at play in relational work. Here Justice explains the Four I's in the way that he would facilitate or teach them:

> The first I stands for internal, which is our relationship to oneself that is developed through what we have learned in relation to the other three I's. The second I is interpersonal, which is the relationship we have with others developed by what we have learned about ourselves

and others. The third I is institutional, which is the relationship we have with social and political institutions such as family, religion, education, healthcare, or government to name some. Our relationship to institutions are developed by what we have learned about ourselves in connection to those institutions. And lastly, the fourth I is ideology, which is the lens from which we see ourselves, understand others and the institutions in our lives. Within this framework ideology presents us with the possibilities of transformational change.

When Justice learned this framework, it was presented as the Four I's of Oppression, a great way to understand that how and what we learn about ourselves and others is mediated through institutions that operate with rigid binarized hierarchies, fixed meanings about social identity, and identity politics. The Four I's are rooted in taking action: learning to question and confront what it is that we believe and why begins with ourselves and is the responsibility of each of us.

The historical context of Body Image 4 Justice and the overall visioning is what connected Justice and me and in large part influenced the roots of Rooted Resistance, which I established in 2016 in Tampa, Florida, to reimagine body-work for racialized queer, trans, and nonbinary people in the United States South and in connection with the land. Years prior, BI4J was gaining more visibility in the greater Boston area due to the extended workshops hosted by Justice at Mike's Fitness in Jamaica Plain for the queer and trans community, namely coaches, massage therapists, and bodyworkers who were working with trans bodies. During this time, I was living in Amherst, Massachusetts, and was seeking to be in community with Black queer and trans people. Through both a Facebook and Google search I found an interview video clip posted by the Boston Neighborhood Network News (BNN). In August 2013 the BNN had aired an interview between news host Chris Lovett and Justice,[2] centered around the Body Image 4 Justice first annual LGBTQAI+ Health and Wellness Weekend, which was co-sponsored by the Hispanic Black Gay Coalition, Massachusetts Transgender Political Coalition, Queer Asian Pacific Asian Alliance, and Mass Equality, among others. Thinking back to this moment, my initial reaction to finding this video clip was joy filled. I remember viewing the clip and nodding along, saying to myself "that's right, that's right." I was overwhelmed with emotion because I had finally found someone in the area who was speaking to my experiences and creating new possibilities. Justice was a lifeline for me. He affirmed for me that continuing to incorporate embodied movement and other forms of healing touch healthcare in my life was a birthright, that I belonged in bodywork spaces, and that such resources were acts of kindness and love for my body. I contacted Justice almost immediately through a Facebook personal message, and shortly after we connected in person in Boston. We have been in each other's lives ever since.

From that point on we started collaborating more through grant writing to secure funding for BI4J. Justice and several BI4J members attended educational workshops in western Massachusetts that would help us expand our network and knowledge. By March 2014 we made an announcement that Body Image 4 Justice, under Black trans and nonbinary leadership, was expanding to western Massachusetts, specifically in Springfield. In the subsequent summer Justice continued to travel to different conferences such as the Philadelphia Trans Health Conference, the National Black Trans Advocacy Conference, FitCom, and the Trans Bodybuilding Competition, where he met Ilya Parker, Noori Jerrard, Sahleem Israel, Rell Freeman, and Preston T. Martin, which began our connection and support as a possible team.

A January 2016 Justice Bodies Collective weekend retreat in North Carolina hosted by Coach Justice brought a group of trans masculine and nonbinary Black people together. It was an oasis to have a safe, intimate, reflective, and supportive environment that ultimately strengthened our collective and encouraged us to continue creating individually. We discussed what the collective vision of Justice Bodies would be moving forward, and we outlined a business plan. Our big initial visioning was to open a gym that was led by and centered around Black queer, trans, nonbinary people. We sought to create a model of what embodied inclusive fitness can look like in our communities. Immediately following the retreat, we collectively launched a fundraising campaign centered on our overarching goal of funding a gym. Simultaneously, Ilya, Roc, and Justice continued to do work in our home state locations.

Decolonizing Fitness (formerly known as Forseca Fitness) is an online educational resource for coaches, trainers, and studio owners established by a Black trans person, Ilya, in memory of his good friend "Big J" Forseca, who passed away of lung cancer. He was transgender, chronically ill, and disabled. He was also cash poor and could not afford most of the medical care he needed living in North Carolina. When he was able to access medical care, he often dreaded going to the doctor because he experienced so much discrimination. Sadly, this is the story of many queer and trans people living in the South, and especially those of us who are located in rural areas across the United States. As Ilya writes on Decolonizing Fitness:

> As someone who personally suffers from chronic hypertension which has now begun to compromise my kidney function, I have experienced firsthand medical discrimination with trying to find trans affirming, educated, and weight neutral medical staff. Several doctors have chosen to focus on my gender and body size as opposed to the conditions that I am seeking medical care for which has left me without receiving adequate and compassionate care.

Decolonizing Fitness was birthed from the need for queer, trans, nonbinary chronically ill and disabled folks to have better access to affirming and supportive health, wellness, and fitness services. Decolonizing Fitness is about helping people develop celebratory, safe, and sustainable movement practices, and providing consultation services to businesses, organizations, and fitness facilities that are interested in improving their accessibility and diversity. Ilya's vision is to assist trans people who want to use movement and training to enable their bodies to more accurately reflect their true selves. Unfortunately, so many vulnerable populations cannot afford or are afraid to access medical providers. Incorporating education and services that will at least aid folks along their path of feeling better in their bodies, Ilya uses his lived experiences, skills, and knowledge from working in the medical industry to create space for people who are often overlooked and devalued.

Justice continued work through BI4J and Justice Bodies in Boston and had the grand opening at his small studio Garage Gym in Hyde Park, Massachusetts. This Garage Gym was specifically created to provide community and fitness support for trans, nonbinary, and gender queer community members.

Justice facilitated individual and group workout training sessions through a sliding scale or free specifically for trans people who did not feel comfortable in gyms and wanted an environment to feel comfortable in their bodies. Garage Gym would end up being the foundation of Justice's Queer Gym Pop Up, which gained national attention on National Public Radio (NPR) in the fall of 2019.[3]

We are determined to expand the programmatic components of each of our services into a fitness curriculum and certification program that seeks to transform oppressive practices in fitness, health, and wellness to be embodied healing justice practices. While this is no simple task, we believe in beginning at the premise that fitness, health, and wellness organizations that employ bodyworkers and practitioners alike have a responsibility to their participants and clients. They need a level of awareness and political analysis regarding how body-image struggles affect people across identities, how people internalize such harmful messages about the body, and how commonplace these issues are.

Creating Fitness 4 All Bodies

In mainstream fitness and coaching environments, there is a prominent white, cisgender, and masculinist network of people, such as Mike Boyle and Dan John, who promote a hegemonic ideology around strength, conditioning, and sport performance.* These modalities are facilitated and taught by promoting a prescribed set of binarized Eurocentric standards that are placed on all bodies to be "fit" and "well" with the particularities of anti-Blackness at the root of their decision making. Trainers, coaches, fitness instructors, and gym and studio owners are some of the gatekeepers of the fitness-industrial

---

* Justice attended the three-day Perform Better Functional Training Summit in July 2015, which provided trainers and coaches educational opportunities and hands-on learning experiences with people in the fitness industry. The workshops were led by able-bodied white cis men and women. The environment and curriculum maintained hypermasculinst values and perpetuated conformity to the gender binary, including trans erasure through instruction.

complex. The very people who have the ability to make significant organizational, facility, personnel, and policy changes within their operations oftentimes do not believe in the value of the radical transformation and change—yet change would make their approaches to "health" and "wellness" more accessible and connected to the lived experiences that people have in their bodies. In part this is due to the commercialization of fitness, exercise, health, and wellness—brand and name recognition are seemingly connected to a particular consumer status. We have observed this within the fitness industry and certification programs. While there are a wide range of personal and group certifications and specializations available, only a few usually get tossed around within the fitness world. Some examples are the National Academy of Sports Medicine, the American Council on Exercise, and the International Sports Sciences Association. We believe this is illustrative of an elitist hierarchy within the fitness, exercise, health, and wellness industry, where people associate certification programs with a spectrum of rigor and status.

Thus, Fitness 4 All Bodies (F4AB) was developed as a collective of trans, queer, and nonbinary trans people who are organizers and educators engaged in racial and gender justice in fitness, sport, and physical culture. Prior to the COVID-19 pandemic we hosted the first Fitness 4 All Bodies panel discussion in Boston. Since then, we have developed a Fitness 4 All Bodies virtual webinar panel series that engages trainers, coaches, body practitioners, and gym owners who are seeking to challenge whiteness and anti-Blackness in the images and ideas associated with our bodies. Panel discussions and live one-on-one chats range from topics such as a training for coaches, using sorties to eradicate toxic masculinity in fitness culture, deconstructing fitness through reclaiming our bodies, embracing our strength because strong is for everybody, and a movement toward healing and resistance led by Black women, Black trans women, and femme embodied nonbinary bodies in the fitness industry. Our webinar series requires critical reflection about the root causes of why we create space, coach, and train in the ways that we do.

Sustaining this work requires both individual and collective commitment and can lead to transformation change and organizational and institutional culture revitalizations. We are struggling far beyond the present for the future possibilities of what the inclusive fitness movement will be. Our curriculum approach and our embodied practices amount to a paradigm shift that rejects capitalist ways of being—the competitive-advantage approach is not what inspires us. Rather, we embrace what we feel as our social and cultural responsibility to develop interventions within our communities that address systemic and institutional oppression in fitness, health, and wellness. Additionally, we share our personal narratives and experiences to create a more inclusive culture at a trainer's or coach's gym or training studio.

A Massachusetts Department of Public Health study comparing LGBTQI+ health with heterosexual and non-transgender counterparts found that trans people had worse outcomes with respect to self-reported health, disability status, anxiety, suicide ideation, and lifetime violence victimization.[4] Our lives are not disposable, and we know that queer and trans people's experiences around health and wellness have been silenced in our society. Body Image 4 Justice seeks to improve such horrific and unacceptable outcomes for queer and trans people through community building and wellness services.

Our work is rooted in transforming the world by debunking both mythical and internalized notions of fitness and bodies. Our ethnographic narrative approach locates "the body" through giving presence to our subjugated identities and experiences within different fitness, medical, and sporting environments. Our collective supports coaches and fitness professionals in developing and refining their social justice lens and critical understanding of diverse and gender-variant bodies in their work, while addressing exclusion and discrimination at the individual and organization levels within the fitness and health industries. We draw on physical cultural studies and Healing Justice to further centralize our work, which is grounded in and narrated through our lived experiences as Black trans men, transmasculine, and nonbinary people who are forced to engage with oppressive social institutions that seemingly promote health and wellness.

Our collective commitment to creating liberatory fitness and healing movement spaces has also been predicated on personal and lived experiences as a praxis to body liberation for transgender, nonbinary, and gender nonconforming people. Our work addresses both the ideology of oppression in the fitness industry, as well as the institutional frameworks that maintain and perpetuate oppression through policy and the privatization of the health industry inclusive of fitness, sport, recreation, and leisure sectors. We offer that our experiences and narratives not only will expand Trans Studies as a field of inquiry but will contribute to the extent in which Black Trans life is conceptualized and theorized as foundational to the understanding of social relations and importantly creating new expansive social relations through such inquiries. Our anthology uses personal stories and experiences to expand understandings of the body and embodied movement through fitness, health, and well-being broadly.

For instance, Ilya Parker's Decolonizing Fitness is more than practicing anti-racism and de-centering Western standards. Instead, engaging with the word *decolonizing* is grounded in the belief that land, power, money, and resources should be returned to the hands of Indigenous Peoples.[5] My project Rooted Resistance centers on reimagining space for queer and trans racialized people in the United States South through embodied movement on the land as a form of healing liberation. Not only is this approach a refusal to commercialized notions of the body, but the premise of Rooted Resistance is predicated on the belief that our bodies and beings are worthy of freedom praxis. Each of us works to address the ideology of oppression in the sport and fitness industry through foundations of grassroots community-based interventions that promote body liberation, racial and gender justice, and a nontoxic culture. Our approach is built through Black feminists' cooperative foundations, such that the personal is political, which allows us to reimagine the ways in which trans people interact with socially constructed and restricted visions of fitness, exercise health, and wellness spaces. As such, we recover imaginative possibilities through a liberatory praxis.

Our shared identities and life experiences have led us to conceptualizing our internal representations of the world and how they affect our external approaches to centering trans community, sharing knowledge through dialogue and the body. This culminative project is well over a decade's worth of reimagining what Justice Roe Williams describes as "activism being rooted in connectivity . . . Connectivity to the self and to others."

Body Image 4 Justice was created because Justice felt that body image was a great connector in regard to people's lived experiences. A more locally focused Body Image 4 Justice has evolved into Fitness 4 All Bodies, an organization and movement that is growing nationally and internationally. A part of our collective power is opening up space for dialogue and discussion about how we see our bodies in ways that challenge toxic ideas we have internalized about ourselves. In other words, refusing the institutional and naturalized ideas about our bodies, gender, and masculinity, we create new, more in-depth ways of being, understanding, celebrating, and loving ourselves and each other. Through dialogue we begin to recognize that our experiences are not always unique solely to our individual selves; rather, they are comprised of interrelated oppressive patterns and institutional practices that are not siloed experiences for trans people. Through this process of unearthing internalized oppression, our narratives make it easier to express to the larger community and society the ways in which we have internalized these ideas about our bodies and that we are reclaiming our truths.

Fitness 4 All Bodies' purpose is centered around making sure that Black trans community members not only had a fitness space to belong, but a space to discuss and heal through unresolved experiences that are often internalized. We centered the specific needs of our overall vitality. Centralizing the body encapsulates the social construction of race, gender, sexuality, disability, nation of origin, ethnicity, and language, to name some. Each part of our fleshy bodies is conceptualized through social and cultural relations, and in this case institutions and organizations that provide healthcare services. Physical cultural studies situate the social significance of (dis)embodied physical culture as having ongoing consequential social and cultural effects both structurally and institutionally.[6] We observe and experience this within the fitness, exercise, health, sport, and wellness industries broadly, whereas reinforcements of Eurocentric racial, gendered, and body hierarchies are commonplace in physical education curriculum including standardized testing, fitness certification trainings, programming, sporting practices, and commercialized gyms and studios.

The Storytelling in This Book

As we proceed, we would like to honor that the words *fitness, health, leisure,* and *wellness* are antithetical to the social institutions that we are forced to engage in within society. We recognize the range of feelings that can surface for people who have historically been told and shown that their bodies do not belong or cannot exist in these spaces as they are. The process of shifting this paradigm in fitness and health must be an ongoing practice.

This anthology is about both honoring the roots of this work and about combining all our contributions to the inclusive fitness movement. The first section, "Ideology: The Ideas and Beliefs We Have Formed around Bodies," seeks to make explicit the learned ideas about our bodies, knowing that making these narratives explicit is the first step toward challenging and transforming them. This is first accomplished by Justice Roe Williams himself defining the concept of the "fitness-industrial complex" in Chapter 1. The fitness-industrial complex acts as the framing lens for the work of Fitness 4 All Bodies with the purpose of making explicit how the fitness industry is both product and perpetuator of white supremacist logic of the body. In Lawrence Koval's piece, "Unknowing the Gym: Moving toward Imagination as Liberation," they examine the origins of the gym as a historically politicized site that manufactures a cisgender, white, heterosexual, and masculinist system—building bodies to labor in service to the nation. Koval explores how gym culture perpetuates the performance of masculinity and femininity as belonging to one gender and structurally advances narrow ideas pathologizing fatness, Blackness, and disability. Unknowing the gym can lead to unveiling the links between the ways that carceral systems are constructed and the construction of gyms and how people move through gyms that oftentimes get chalked up to be "leisurely" spaces of escape.

In M Camellia's piece, "My Body, Anarchy," they explore agency and motivations within the realm of the physical body, employing the lens of yogic philosophy in an accessible way. These ideas are contextualized within tenets of informed and enthusiastic consent that are typically related solely to the realm of sexuality, applying them to contemporary fitness/wellness culture and our internal and external work to liberate our individual and collective bodies. Through personal narrative, Camellia reflects on their own experiences as a fat, Trans, and chronically ill person who is also continually recovering from disordered eating and exercise. Within that shell, the piece looks at the ways dominant culture currently drives modern fitness culture from a position of external authority, re-creating itself on increasingly micro scales until it's embedded in our tissues, and weaponizing our minds against our already-oppressed bodies as a means of perpetuating the white supremacist, capitalist status quo.

Beyond examining how systems of oppression are internalized and mirrored within our industries, businesses, models, fitness/wellness classes and services, and our bodies and behaviors, this essay also seeks to put forth potential balms. Among them are self-inquiry practices that investigate external sources of motivation with respect to our physical bodies (think inaccessibility/gatekeeping, hierarchical fitness, yoga class structures, "fitspo," desirability politics, etc.) and aid in reorientation toward an innate desire for liberation and the accompanying responsibilities; a framework of de-vilified pleasure, particularly for those facing systemic oppression, that reframes it as a vital litmus test to gauge our desire and connect us to our personal agency; and examples of what a broader personal consent praxis can offer us collectively in the near term.

Our second section, "Personal Experiences with Others and Institutions," gives our community members space to share how the fitness-industrial complex has created personal experiences and been enacted upon the body. John R. Bridger begins with "Push-Ups and Privilege," depicting a story of a little rural Alaskan kid with hoop dreams who grew up understanding the necessity of collective community care. Now a mental health practitioner who finds solace in the weight room, Bridger had introspection that led him to recognize how he often masked his athlete identity to distance himself from manifestations of white patriarchal masculinity embedded within fitness culture. Recognizing the shame that accompanied his cisgender, white, tall, able-bodied privilege, Bridger started living a compartmentalized life until finding community members online who were probing and reframing their masculinity. Learning to challenge the foundations of toxic masculinity and commercial weight training spaces have shifted his relationship to self and the internalized belief that vulnerability and care are characteristics that men did/could not embody. Individual stories are in relationship to structural forces, which can shift our ability to both know and love ourselves. In her essay "Learning to Love My Body beyond Perception," Adele Jackson-Gibson critically addresses layers of other perceptions on her physicality, further contextualizing these experiences through the enclosure of whiteness and the rigid notions of what it means to be a Black queer woman who is athletic. Reclaiming her story through a reflexive examination of racial and gendered physicality, this piece uncovers the harm associated with pushing the body to the limit and rediscovers boundaries through integrative restorative practices. Noticing, listening to the body, being still, and being immersed in a community of care can transform the way we think and act toward the body—moving toward a more loving relationship with ourselves is a window into the inextricability of our connectedness.

In the final section of this anthology, "How We Empowered Ourselves to Move Forward and Help Our Communities Polish Their Armor," we get insight into what hopes, dreams, and visions exist when it comes to creating fitness rooted in philosophies of care and healing. We are living in a time when trans and gender variant folks are more visible than ever, yet trans folks are still being violently targeted by people in their own communities. Many of us trans individuals are forced to hide who we are in order to remain safe. Trans, queer, and gender diverse people need to be in physical and virtual spaces where we are met with compassion. We need to be encouraged and supported when we engage in movement practices that allow for us to embrace all of who we are.

Asher Freeman's essay "Landmines" arises from using weight lifting as a way to come into their body and begin addressing years of gender dysphoria. Their story begins after losing their dream job and learning how enmeshed their identity had become with paid work. As they stepped into their life as an unemployed person, the physical and emotional discomforts that had been previously overshadowed by busy work life became too loud to ignore. This follows their journey through fitness, facing uncomfortable truths about their body, and onto forging their path as a personal trainer with the goal of sharing their own learning with others who feel a similar disconnect between their body and mind.

Connecting the body in an integrative and a communal way takes shape in Sonja R. Price Herbert's "Reframing Pilates to Meet Our Bodies," where she explores her racialized gender as a Black woman in fitness spaces. Experiencing patterns of erasure within the Pilates community, in 2017 she created Black Girl Pilates, an organization that centers sisterhood through movement. In "Fitness of the Soul," Sunaina Rangnekar situates us in the reshaping of their approach as a yoga practitioner—centering queer and nonbinary experiences and knowledge while honoring their whole being as a part of the global majority. Unsettling the soul—the erasure, exploitation, and commodification of the cultural and historical roots of yoga through Western disruptions of this sacred practice—led to an accountability process to address the harm and embody an ethical practice. Rangnekar extends to us practical ways to do internal work through prompt writing and reflection.

Similar questions are posed in Beck Beverage's "On Leaving the Fitness-Industrial Complex," where they document their experience as a studio owner, trying to push back against the confines of the fitness industry, and ultimately their decision to step away from fitness toward a different approach and philosophy of movement practice. They share how they work with clients now outside of the definitions of fitness, the space they created, and how compensation plays into this work. In Dr. Marcia Dernie's piece, "Embracing the Body After Change," they share their narrative around coming into their body in movement and strength training. From early days at the YMCA to powerlifting competitions, diet culture, the medical industrial complex, loss, grief, disability, and a resurgence of nourishing forms of movement, this piece captures the dehumanizing and institutionalized scope of ableism and the manufactured guilt and shame that is both placed on and internalized within the body. By less "powering through" and more reframing movement expectations in relation to our body's wisdom, we can find pathways to liberation.

In connection to loss and grief, Damali Fraiser's "The Body as a Site of Oppression and Freedom" centers layers of Damali's life story as a Black Caribbean Canadian woman and kettlebell coach. She contextualizes her experiences practicing Muay Thai, her relationship with food, and with movement later on in life. As a survivor of gender-based violence, Damali thought that the physicality and skill of this martial arts resonated with her need to protect herself and her children. However, Damali's physical body was probed by outsiders, leading to an obsession regarding her weight loss and body aesthetic. The notion of treating our bodies with noncare within the realms of fitness and body movement is a gateway to maintaining disembodied experiences that shift us further away from our bodies. Damali expresses that Black fitness professionals are actively refusing this notion by creating space for continued learning and collective healing.

Continuing this thread of transformation from the personal to political, Kanoelani Patterson writes "How My Fatness Helped Me Reclaim My Power and Tell My Story," where she looks back on her life to realize how much she went through to become the woman she is today and how she is empowered to be someone to encourage her community toward liberation, growth, and continuing to nourish themselves in all that they are and will become. She draws upon her experience growing up as a Fat Black girl in mostly white, thin spaces, making it almost impossible for her to ever feel like she was enough, leading to her developing many insecurities, traumas, and mental health issues. Through the combination of fatphobia, racism, and diet culture, she was always on a diet—a common phenomenon for a lot of Fat folx. She reflects on her experience being put on a diet in fourth grade at the age of ten. After struggling through diet culture, eating disorders, and mental health issues such as depression, anxiety, panic attacks, and suicidal ideation, her brightest hope is that someone can see what she's been through and realize they are not alone in their journey in life. There are many people just like them dealing with oppressive systems and finding ways, in spite of them all, to flourish and thrive—not just survive their trauma, but truly live full lives that they richly deserve.

Finally, Rebby Kern's personal essay "Moving from Allyship to Solidarity" is a reflection of their journey as a Black trans, nonbinary, adopted, disabled, queer yoga teacher activating a community of comrades who commit to their unlearning and solidarity to communities who are pushed away from fitness and wellness space. They share the impacts of their national race and gender bias workshops, how community commitment shifts and grows following ongoing violence toward the transgender and BIPOC communities and how tangible change has been implemented in these spaces. Upon entering the yoga and wellness world, they quickly discovered that their Black, trans, and queer identities were not reflected in studio culture. While engaging in their practice, they helped co-found the Trans Yoga Project, a national collective of trans and nonbinary yoga and wellness leaders across the US who are working together to uplift the experiences and talents of trans and queer yoga teachers, educate studio leadership on affirming spaces, and disrupt the status quo by honoring decolonizing practices in these spaces. The impact of their work moves people from fragility to action-oriented solidarity, uplifting and honoring the voices and experiences of trans yoga teachers and students.

Through these personal narratives, this anthology seeks to begin the explicit naming of what constitutes the fitness-industrial complex, how it has harmed us, and how to dismantle it. But like most radical work, this is not simply a destructive process, but one that promises to build something new. These new ways of relating to fitness need not be perfect. But they are rooted in the firm belief that what currently exists is inherently untenable—and that we are envisioning new worlds and bringing them into practice.

PART I

Ideology:
The Ideas and Beliefs We Have Formed around Bodies

CHAPTER 1

The Foundation of This Space Is Love

JUSTICE ROE WILLIAMS

At First My Life Was Musical

I am a poet. I am my mother's child. I am so many things that deserve equal acknowledgement and celebration. Coming to understand life first through the eyes of my mother, then through the eyes of society, and finally through my own eyes, I recognize that my calling was to become both a connector and a movement maker. Simple snapshots of my life reflect courage, resilience, and the opportunities to grow from my many mistakes. I think about my middle school experience of being isolated because I learned differently than the other students and was placed in special education classes. Then how I went on to graduate high school in the top 20 of my class. I was a part of the National Honor Society during both my junior and senior years. It's like when someone says I can't do something, I make sure that I do and that they know it. It's these images that create the frame of who I am today and why I am so passionate about working with my community and moving toward liberation.

I was born in Atlantic City, New Jersey, in 1974. This was during the dissipation of the Black Power movement—a movement I would not learn about until my first year of college. To me, this sounded like the smooth vibrations of "Could It Be I'm Falling in Love" by the Spinners, "We Are Family" by Sister Sledge, "(If Loving You Is Wrong) I Don't Want to Be Right" by Luther Ingram, and my father's favorite, "After the Love Has Gone" by Earth, Wind & Fire. This became the ballad of my father leaving our lives. This impacted me greatly because I was "daddy's little girl," after all. My childhood felt regular. It was full of love, laughter, joy, play, but it was then I realized that my dark skin made me less worthy. Even though we were all living in the same place, I knew I was lesser than. I was always picked on and bullied. I felt shame, anger, and sometimes worthlessness.

Body image became an important factor to me after puberty. There was no language to help me understand my feelings. I suffered silently thinking I was so far from God. I was constantly praying for deliverance. It wasn't the church that delivered me, it was what my mom created right at home. Church was home with "No Charge" by Shirley Caesar, "I Don't Feel No Ways Tired" by Rev. James Cleveland, "Lost without You" by BeBe and CeCe Winans, and Mom's favorite, "Precious Lord, Take My Hand" by Mahalia Jackson. The more I prayed, the more I heard nothing but silence. And even the music that had held me began to fade as I moved away from my mother's arms into a world that could amputate me and throw me away.

Always Jumping into and out of Boxes

In both my life and my activism, I have always been asked to separate my identities and prioritize which fight is most important to me. When I felt silenced in one community, I would find another and still feel disconnected within it. I felt like I always had to put on the performance of normalcy. Growing up, I felt this drive to connect even though I had always been pushed into separating the pieces of my identity. This separation is a tool of a white supremacist culture, or a culture of the colonized that has been used as a weapon against bodies throughout time.

Growing up I felt overwhelmed by the conflict I felt inside myself. I believe one of the hard things about body image is that we give other people authority to define who we are and determine our worth. I internalized negative ideas about being Black, about being a Black woman, about being queer, about my transition, about being a Black man, and how all of this connects to the ways that I move both in my body and in the world. I internalized so much conflict from the messages I received about my body growing up, I never understood that I would be able to break free from the chains of my performance of gender in relation to sexuality and being Black.

I never understood that "freedom" was wearing whiteness in black skin, and what that meant about how I valued myself. I jumped in and out of boxes. This performance made me feel safe and allowed me certain "freedoms." What I was learning about myself in that white face was self-hate under the guise of feeling valued. We are all in search of the "American Dream" that says we deserve "God's gifts," but only if you are white, cisgender, heterosexual, male, possess capital, and have an able body to get you there. In these lies we all exist, and inside I knew this performance was killing me slowly.

What I learned about my body didn't feel true in the ways that a caterpillar is just a caterpillar. I was born into black skin and tossed into pink pajamas to parents living below the poverty line. I was my mother's daughter and daddy's little girl, but to me I just was. I existed in all of the ways until that identity limited the way that I saw my own Blackness and who I could be in this body. To the world, I was some poor Black family's little girl. I was nothing and, as a result, I erased my body and how I experienced my body. Much like Pinocchio, I became a puppet not living but performing in this body.

Throughout my childhood and into my adulthood, I conformed to ideas and existed in ways that were not true. I turned to self-destructive behaviors as a means to numb the pain of erasure. I believed I was the problem, and this was reinforced by my parents, church, school, and what I saw on TV. The options for poor Black children during the '70s and '80s were limited to the service industry, sports, or entertainment, and then the lucky ones who got out of the ghetto. I now see this as the foundation for my need to exist in a collective as a whole community. I now know that what I was told does not have to be the truth. This idea became my cocoon of trust and began the process of changing the narrative in my life.

I Believe in the Power of Connection

In the early '90s, I found more than my voice. I found collective power. It was during college that I was able to actively find a community that embraced me just as I was—or that's how it felt at the time. I was surrounded by and in community with some amazing activists from across the United States who were connected to former Black Panthers, former members of the Young Lords Party, and MOVE members, and we also joined with Indigenous activists working for Free Leonard Peltier. I was in my early twenties, and in a way I felt we were romanticizing the successes of past movements and not finding new strategies to combat injustice. We rallied, protested, and rebelled. I had my share of impromptu missions to drop banners or wheat-paste flyers. This was an extremely radical time in my life because I felt rage from years of being told I wasn't enough and "this is just the way it is." So I was on fire.

This set into motion my understanding of the power of the collective. It also showed me how whiteness has a way to infiltrate any space even if there is not one white person in the room. I say this because some four or five years later, I felt used and silenced experiencing sexism for being perceived as a woman, homophobia, and, please, let's not discuss the conversations I had around gender identity. I found myself not just having to compromise my morals and values, but being totally erased as if I wasn't there at all. This is a historical cycle of erasure of queer, trans, and disabled Black bodies. If it wasn't valued by whiteness, it was not deemed valuable in our smaller community. Therefore, the struggle was not as much about equality but being valued in a culture that says "Black lives don't matter," so the only fight to be had was about being Black.

Even when I moved to Boston while doing political prisoner work or any activism within the Black community, it was not okay for me to express or discuss being trans or queer. I felt that the narrative about my gender was dictated by those around me, and conforming meant I would be both respected and not demonized by those I was in connection with. In the communities I was a part of during the late '90s, we were not talking about gender or sexuality in the ways we do today. So even during that activism, my body, which was perceived as that of a very strong woman, was often used violently against the male-identified members of the group. I would be used as an example of strength, and male-identified members would be emasculated and shamed for not being as strong as me. In the movement for Black liberation, we all had to be strong since we knew we were up against violence, but women were not supposed to be stronger than men.

In the mid to late '90s—heck, even today—Boston was a very segregated town. At first it was hard for me to navigate. I moved in with my cousin who lived in Malden, which at that time was largely white, and I rarely saw Black folks where I lived. I had to make my daily trips to Roxbury, which felt more like home to me and was where I was able to connect with queer Black artists, poets, activists, and youth workers. I felt myself distancing myself from political prisoner work because I could no longer silence myself. I decided I needed to find ways to change what activism looks like, and working with youth was my answer. Youth work connected me to the powerful process of meeting people where they are at and seeing that it takes a village to raise a child. It impressed upon me the need to move together as a community to create change. In my work with young people, I found myself in circles with Christians, politicians, and youth development directors from agencies across greater Boston.

In the late '90s the trans community was raging. I could not continue to watch Black trans women dying. When Rita Hester died in '98,[1] I was distraught. I was working at a job where my supervisor would misgender me on a regular basis, and I had just been a part of a youth conference where I was outed in front of a larger audience of youth workers. There simply was no care or respect for the contributions of trans people to our larger community, and I had enough. So I followed my purpose and I became a connector.

In 1998 I organized what was known as the Truth Rally, which served as a point of connection and opened so many doors for the trans community in Boston. I used my body as the glue to bring the different communities together to march and protest media misrepresentation. This rally had participation from communities that don't normally engage with each other, like the Jericho Committee (Organization to Free Political Prisoners), Workers

World Party (Boston Socialist Movement), the National Committee to Free Puerto Rican Political Prisoners, SOUL (Students Organizing for Unity and Liberation), Queer Revolt, A Slice of Rice, the Lesbian Avengers, MOCAA, and others. I remember the energy of building with communities that I was a part of and feeling all in one moment, acknowledging all of who I am. The rally was a learning experience for all. We were able to unite under one issue that affects us all: the media.

I believe in the power of the collective. Even though that coalition did not stay together, it reminded me again that there is power in connection. This coalition helped inspire other activists to step up and create agencies to support trans communities that still exist today. It also inspired the annual National Transgender Day of Remembrance, held in memorial to remember the lives of trans individuals who have died from structural violence against our community.

After my transition, I began building a community for the transmasculine-identified community in Boston. I was doing consulting work with different nonprofits in Boston and decided to start a nonprofit called Body Image 4 Justice (BI4J). The work of BI4J was to bring movement, health, and wellness to bodies that were not welcome to gyms, healthcare centers, hospitals, and mental health providers. Our core value was: "We believe that a positive body image and self-esteem are the foundation of health and that there is no wrong way to have a body." I was doing a lot of research and having community discussions about the issues we faced being trans people of color living in Boston. This work grew through collaborations with activists who lived in Springfield, Massachusetts, and with youth organizations in Boston.

Much of the challenge was dealing with a very racist and transphobic queer community, including those who provide LGBTQ mental health and wellness services in Boston. In response, BI4J held monthly conversations for trans people of color, social justice workshops for those who were body practitioners like fitness coaches and massage therapists, and we partnered with the local sex shop, which provided us with packers that were made for men of color, binders, and condoms and lube. We organized the first transmasculine show-and-tell for top surgery support and partnered with Community Kinship Life, a trans organization in New York, to sponsor the first transfeminine show-and-tell. These were a way for people to share their top surgery results and talk about the process from start to finish. BI4J became a space for our bodies to be loved just as they are, and that love was carried into the work of Fitness 4 All Bodies.

Beyond Accessorization and Accommodations

In 2012 I began working at a gym as their front desk person, around the corner from where I lived. I honestly got the job because it was the closest gym and I could not afford the membership. I was also working as the trans navigator at the Queer Health Center in Boston and still actively creating spaces for connection and conversation within the trans communities of color. I started working out regularly at the gym, bringing my friends who identified as trans into the gym, and showing them how to use the weights and how to approach the gym when they don't feel safe. One of the trainers asked if I was interested in working as a trainer on their team, and that invitation brought in a new wave of activism.

At our gym, I was the only trans-identified trainer, and I am going to say with no hesitation that I was also the queerest person employed at our facility. I not only became pretty significant in maintaining a space of joy and creating a sense of belonging, but I also served like security in the way that I was always kicking somebody out of spaces for being disgusting toward women or discriminatory toward the trans members. Sometimes my job simply included helping trans folks feel comfortable using whichever dressing room suited them, as our facility did not have gender-neutral options. To be honest, even my clients who did not identify as trans did not feel comfortable in gyms. I began to ask what social justice looks like in our movement spaces.

In 2013 I took over the gym and held the first annual LGBTQ Health and Wellness Weekend. I wanted to put some theory into practice for all of the pieces of the work I have done within our smaller fitness community. During the weekend, we changed the smaller employee restroom into a gender-neutral restroom, and we had conversations with members about etiquette in spaces, especially the shower area and dressing rooms. Of course, this was not a one-time conversation; it was a part of my daily ritual to push the members' boundaries around community and gender. All the program staff who taught group classes worked with me on creating space for all bodies. We also had conversations about body image and identity. This showed me that we can make space for all bodies in a community that is still learning and moving away from hate.

After some time as a coach, I wanted to try and expand this ideology that movement belongs to all using the experience I had gained in doing this work. The result was Queer Gym Pop Up, a movement space centering love, at a small studio in Brookline, Massachusetts, and then expanded briefly in Dorchester. Queer Gym Pop Up is not rooted in a hypermasculine ideology around strength and movement. We started by creating community agreements that were visible to everyone in the space. Everyone had the opportunity to add to our agreements. People felt welcomed. It's funny, what I think of when everyone enters the space is the *Cheers* intro when it says everybody knows your name. It was true. We knew everybody's name, and in everyone's own way we all connected.

I integrated the work of BI4J with the Pop Up. The result was movement sessions, healing discussions, dinner nights, and having a space to chill, relax, and be in community. All of this programming was donation-based. Queer Gym Pop Up received a lot of attention from local and national news. Previously, queer community gyms were not welcoming spaces for everyone. The Pop Up welcomed the larger community. There was fear that if we welcomed everyone, it would become just like any other gym. We were able to show that movement spaces can be for all bodies without being like other gyms. When people walk through the door and we know their name, they know they are part of something larger and more authentic.

Putting All the Pieces Together

From high school to present day, the gym has been a central part of my life—even throughout my activism. It was a constant reflection of my relationship to my body. I found my physical strength through the gym, and it became a way to be in community with bodies that I felt aligned with. However, being in the gym was a constant reminder that I was not viewed as a man. So the gym was not a space where I belonged. Even though my experience had been alienating and dehumanizing, I made space for my body by conforming to hyperaggressive, dominating ideas of masculinity. I later challenged these ideas and unlearned the way I had been taught to view my body. Instead, I had to accept all of who I am. This process of unlearning happens daily. I question whether something feels authentic to me and how I want to experience love.

Now, whenever I think about the relationships I create in community with others, I often think about the Four I's of Oppression framework, which Roc mentioned in the book's introduction. I have used this as a tool to assess the impact of oppression on my own life and to teach others how to examine dominant narratives of othering and its impact on our bodies and our lives. What I find most important about this framework is that it gives a clear understanding that the 4 I's (internal, interpersonal, institutional, and ideological) cannot exist separately. This means that in our work to eradicate oppression, we must challenge oppression at all four levels. Body image—how we are taught to view and be in relationship to our bodies—is an ideology that we must deconstruct using this framework. When we begin to see how body image is used as a tool by white supremacist culture, specifically to mold us into productive citizens, we recognize our connectedness as a larger community, and social change happens.

As a fitness coach, I have always been engaged in discussions about body image, and in each conversation, a connection was made about what we had learned from toxic fitness culture. Ilya Parker explains this perfectly on his website Decolonizing Fitness:

> Social characteristics, language and habits that promote/reinforce ableism, fatphobia, racism, classism, elitism, body shaming/policing, LGBTQIA+ hatred under the guise of fitness and wellness.

> Toxic fitness culture relies on two distinct groups to be situated on opposite ends of the fitness spectrum. One group consists of the non-disabled, thin/toned, [conventionally] attractive, young,

cisgender, heterosexual people who are assumed to be the gatekeepers of what it means to engage appropriately in & embody fitness.[2]

Everyone I have met feels like their body needed to be fixed. Losing weight, being more toned, it all means wanting to be desired by a society that values standards that nobody can meet or maintain.

As a larger community, we are all jumping into and out of the boxes that whiteness places us in. Whiteness separates us from ourselves and each other through its desire to define and prescribe. Separated, we all fall for the lies that we are told about the bodies of those around us. In all my work I have found that the only way we are going to understand this separation and the intentions behind it is to create spaces where we can expose ourselves to each other. In this we are using our vulnerability to teach and not using the experiences of those who are marginalized to make more space for white bodies. Whiteness is incomprehensible to white people. Their experience of it, therefore, does not allow experiences outside whiteness to be seen as standard, normal, or mainstream, because whiteness dictates what is normal.

We attach ourselves to labels and identities defined for us so that we may find commonality. That could mean or become community, but for me it has felt more like silencing pieces of myself that made those around me feel uncomfortable. Therefore, being in community with anyone has been challenging because I wasn't exposed to the language to share my experience of my body with others. I lived in the shadows of everyone's perceptions of my race, my gender, and the ways that I should move and experience my body.

I do understand this is not my lone experience. When we are separated and divided from our internal identity, it is easy to be molded. It is easy to be lied to. We can no longer exist in movements that model our oppression. bell hooks, American author, professor, and feminist, helps us understand our experience by providing us with the language to understand the interlocking nature of our experiences. I would add to this the interlocking of ideas that we internalize about gender and sexuality to this overarching ideology of dominant culture. hooks tells us that we must think critically about our experiences within that construct, and that this is the only way we can move forward.

These ideas are connected to and framed by how we experience our own body image, which is both a tool of the fitness-industrial complex and a way to have a conversation about oppression and the ideas we hold about bodies. I believe that we have all been lied to about how we should value, experience, and exist in our bodies. Our worth has then been determined by patriarchal whiteness, how it manipulates our identities, and through dictating the ways we live in our bodies.

Author and poet Audre Lorde said it best: "I cannot afford the luxury of fighting one form of oppression only. I cannot afford to believe that freedom from intolerance is the right of only one particular group."[3] I say no more jumping into and out of boxes. No more silencing myself in order to find value. We need to free ourselves from white supremacy acting as a puppeteer and instead expose ourselves to new views and perspectives. We need to find spaces like my cocoon of trust where we can have conflict and become expansive, not limited. We need to embrace conflict as it creates growth, adaptability, and change. This led me to the work and activism of creating spaces for all bodies, because I know my experience of being Black, living in a larger body, being perceived as a Black woman, and as the man I am today. I know what it feels like to be distanced from the comfort of just being me.

I cut the puppet strings, and now I can be authentically myself by acknowledging the ways that I experience the interlocking systems of oppression and naming this injustice. I was inspired by Carol Hanisch's quote "the personal is political,"[4] which sparked a movement rooted in our personal experiences of these systems. My hope is to challenge those within the fitness industry to understand what social justice means within our community movement spaces. I hope to give practitioners a sense of how great of an impact and influence these oppressive social institutions that make up the fitness-industrial complex have been on our movement practice, our clients, and our bodies.

Fitness Is for All Bodies

What began as a day of education and movement has grown into a collective of BIPOC queer, trans, and disabled individuals connected by the idea of fitness being for all bodies. In January 2020 I hosted Fitness 4 All Bodies' first live event at Achieve Fitness in Somerville, Massachusetts. At Achieve, I never felt like I had to conform or hide my identity and felt like it was a place that community could be brought together. The result was a panel featuring the Achieve Fitness staff, Linda Wellness Warrior, Nicolas Hall, and Shawn Garcia of RevFit. During this panel, we shared our personal stories of how we experienced fitness and why we created the spaces we did.

Learning happens when we are able to be vulnerable with each other. We were able to create a space that left the audience in tears over our personal stories and what we were willing to share. People expressed how affirmed they felt, how they wanted more of these spaces, and wondering how to create them. After the morning panel, facilitators led a movement practice in the afternoon. They shared their coaching styles from cueing to sharing modifications and variations of exercises. This helped coaches understand the importance of language and the way of reframing movement that could be affirming to all bodies. It was made clear that being in movement with others is inherently vulnerable and coaches are put in a position of authority over their client's bodies. I believe that for many people attending the event, this was their first time being exposed to these ideas and practices. Their expectations of what fitness could and should be were cracked wide open.

This space was one of connection and imagination, where we could begin to consider what could come next if we considered the way body image and the fitness-industrial complex limit the way we connect with ourselves and each other. I still feel a bit overwhelmed by the impact of this event, especially in contrast to the way the larger world is engulfed in war, constant conflict, and constant fear.

While organizing this event, I was asked to facilitate a similar event at a gym in New York run by the Women's Strength Coalition and a gym in Philadelphia run by someone I connected to during a kettlebell certification. Then the COVID-19 pandemic shifted our world. Many people were forced to confront the realities of the world we live in. The pandemic brought more than death. Depression, fear, and white rage were all given authority from our own president, who was held up by misinformation and propaganda.

Black people were dying at a higher rate than white people. We were hearing more bad news each day. Then the deaths of Ahmaud Arbery in February 2020, Breonna Taylor in March 2020, George Floyd in May 2020, and Tony McDade in June 2020 sparked an awareness and attention to systemic racism and injustice. We had to ask ourselves, do Black lives really matter? The truth is that if we have to ask this question, the answer is no. I was lost in despair being separated from my parents, both of whom are immunocompromised. I worried about their health and safety while I battled the virus myself. I was able to recover without going to the hospital, but had a long two months of recovery.

Being pushed into the virtual world because of the pandemic did make possibilities for connection and creation. Fitness 4 All Bodies was able to collaborate with other fitness spaces virtually and with respected content creators and influencers like Chrissy King, all of whom have been changing the fitness industry in their own ways. Our programming included Black women and femmes discussing their experience in the fitness industry, disabled fitness professionals talking about their experiences of ableism, and monthly discussions with gym owners and fitness professionals about their careers and the spaces they've created.

Due to the positive response to panels, we expanded our programming to include courses and curriculum to counter the narrative of what is often taught in the fitness industry. With the mission of helping fitness professionals hone and use a social justice lens in their work, we taught—and currently offer—courses about masculinity, eugenics, and the intersections of race, gender, ability, class, and fitness. We created this programming by illuminating voices that are often erased and taking the lead from leaders in the margins that are rarely acknowledged. Queer Gym Pop Up also moved to being held virtually and under the Fitness 4 All Bodies umbrella. This is a space where our teachings could be applied and put into action, where people attending could see how cues matter and how to welcome people into a space.

Whether it is an Instagram Live, educational course, panel discussion, or workout, I wanted to continue to provide opportunities for people to see what is possible when we challenge the ways we've been taught to be in our bodies and what can be created from connecting with one another. Even this chapter I am writing I hope can be another opportunity for this purpose.

Our Bodies Are Our Movement

Through the stories and experiences of trainers, coaches, and bodyworkers from different backgrounds, we hope you are able to contextualize the effects of the fitness-industrial complex on all bodies. This is a framework I created to name that fitness, as an industry, acts systemically to both produce and ideologically maintain dominant body cultures. Bringing together these voices of activists within the fitness industry who are deconstructing and re-envisioning how we experience and understand fitness as it presently exists, this book shows the ways in which we are all connected in this fight to redefine fitness as a practice or ritual for all bodies.

The concept of Fitness 4 All Bodies allows all of us to explore and discuss our differences in connection to the larger structures that oppress us by forcing us to conform to white supremacist cis-hetero patriarchal capitalistic ideas. Fitness as a practice has become centered around one's appearance or aesthetic versus defining whole-body wellness for ourselves. This erases the unique needs of the individual, while selling the lie that members of society must meet certain artificial criteria of "health" by any means necessary.

Between social media and traditional forms of media, we are constantly being fed this toxic ideology of not only what it means to be fit but to look fit, much less participate in fitness. We develop damaging beliefs about our own bodies and their acceptability, thus further buying into the idea that the only way to be fit is to be young, lean, and muscular. The fitness-industrial complex thrives on the stigma it creates against bodies that don't meet this standard—that is, the majority of all our bodies.

Redefining Fitness

The fitness-industrial complex defines and maintains power over our bodies through patriarchal, white supremacist culture. These mainstream ideas teach us that the white, cisgender, heterosexual, non-disabled, middle-class, and thin body is the standard that needs to be aspired to in the interest of perpetuating a society based on a social caste system, thus creating the image of the "productive citizen." The fitness-industrial complex is maintained by private companies that make huge profits from diet and fitness culture, given that through white supremacist body culture no one will truly attain these standards, and this failure is required for it to perpetuate. The fitness industry becomes a space to attempt to rehabilitate "non-desirable" bodies, or ones that do not fit the image of the productive citizen, thus damaging our bodies, our relationship to our bodies, and our mental health.

Opposing the monolithic and oppressive ideals upheld by the fitness-industrial complex, the body positivity movement is led by BIPOC disability activists, and it's time that we uplift that narrative. As members of the movement, we challenge the idea that fitness belongs to only one body type and that there is only one way to be fit. Because fitness is for all bodies and the personal is still political, we fight against the false messages and body-shaming beliefs promoted by the fitness-industrial complex.

Today's fight for Fitness 4 All Bodies includes coaches and trainers who are often seen as gatekeepers and spokespeople for the fitness industry. As agents of this industry, we can take action to support our clients and contradict the harmful messages that the industry perpetuates in order to make profit and perpetuate this impossible idea of the "fit body." Even further, we need to deconstruct the fitness-industrial complex by using our own stories and experiences of the fitness industry. In order to eradicate the fitness industry, we must be connected through our differences to build an impenetrable armor to protect us as we change the narrative of what fitness means for all bodies.

Deconstructing the fitness-industrial complex is no easy task. It is not enough to try to amend or accessorize these spaces with missions of "inclusivity" or "diversity." Rather, as activist Roc Rochon of Rooted Resistance shared while participating in the August 2020 Fitness 4 All Bodies panel, we must first recognize the way gym spaces and fitness perpetuate these dynamics on a systemic level, then deconstruct it by building from the ground up spaces that center and prioritize different values such as fat, queer, BIPOC liberation, and disability justice. Fitness 4 All Bodies is not a commodity, but rather a liberation movement for all our bodies.

Planting Seeds

What I have learned from this long journey of activism and loving myself beyond what the world has told me is that I need to plant the following seeds: Belonging, Looking Back (Sankofa), Education, Healing, and Leadership Development. These have become our Seeds of Growth.

Belonging is like a cocoon that holds space for us to engage in conflict in ways that support both unlearning and acceptance of new information. Some may think it's a space where everything is in alignment with our current ideas, beliefs, and values, yet it's a space where we can be at our most vulnerable to expose and be exposed to our authenticity. Belonging is a process where trust happens and we understand that we carry so much pain, hurt, and distrust that it may seem overwhelming to think what it means to create this space through our differences. We start the process of Belonging with communicating and always in communication with what everyone needs in that space.

When I say Looking Back, I mean like Sankofa, which is a word from the Akan tribe in Ghana, Africa, that translates to "it is not taboo to fetch what is at risk of being left behind." When I think about looking back, it is a reckoning to go learn from multiple perspectives to fill in the gaps that whiteness has created. We can't understand ourselves today without looking back at our past. If we are reframing the ways in which we are connecting with ourselves and each other, it's important to understand the roots of who, how, and where we have learned the ideas we hold about ourselves and others. This looking back becomes a needed ritual, a daily process of understanding and examining who we are today.

With Education, we are learning every day through exposure, but what are we being exposed to? How are we framing our education? Who are we learning from about bodies? I believe it is important to illuminate the voices and experiences of communities that have been oppressed, silenced, and erased. Learning and investing in these experiences are just as important as learning about whiteness. I always say learning is easy and should be defined as something that happened for each of us in our own way. It's what we carry and find privilege in holding on to that makes unlearning the toughest task.

Healing is necessary in order for us to trust enough to believe that we can truly be in a space of belonging with those who never wanted to let us in. We have to find space to heal and recover from past trauma that we carry in our bodies from generations of being oppressed, amputated, and tossed away. We live in a world that is constantly policing our bodies and exploiting our experiences, silencing us into erasure. We will never trust if we can't heal, and healing starts when we find that forgiveness is more a selfish act than we may feel.

Leadership Development is a deep process of understanding ourselves and our greater responsibility in bringing community back together. If we continue to look at building relationships with our neighbors as something extra, it costs too much and we will never move from the divide that exists between us. Leadership development is reframing and acknowledging the ways we need to step up and have the courage to change that narrative.

Working within the fitness industry, we need to see ourselves as the change agents. We need to be a sword against the fitness-industrial complex while shielding our clients from toxic fitness culture. You must open yourself up to new information that challenges your current ideologies. One of my favorite coaches, Jason Pak, taught me that "we learn from bodies, not books." This made me more confident in my approach; everything just clicked when I heard it. Accept what we don't know and that we are constantly learning!

We need to prioritize not just learning but listening, healing, looking back, and building our armor, as well. In the work of Fitness 4 All Bodies, this has looked like courses, panels, discussions, all focused on building beyond difference and making these discussions more readily available. We need to learn how to engage with diverse bodies and each other in more authentic, genuine ways. This means deviating from the prescriptive model of whiteness that focuses on fixing the body. Instead, we celebrate the differences in our bodies—both between one another and even our own bodies over time and experience.

When we initiate any community activity with Fitness 4 All Bodies, we ensure two things. The first is a land acknowledgement, as we know that it's just the beginning of the journey toward changing our social narrative around people, place, and history. For Fitness 4 All Bodies, we want to look at the land we inhabit through the lens of its original people, not those of the colonizer. We acknowledge that we are on the land of Massachusetts peoples and that they are the original inhabitants of this land. We ask you to learn about why making a land acknowledgement is important.

Second, we welcome everyone into the space by building a cocoon of trust. This is a list of agreements that we use to remind us of our responsibility toward maintaining a sense of belonging:

1. Trust intent, name impact: As we enter a conversation, we work to trust that the intention is connection while acknowledging the impact we have with our words.

2. Take space, make space: Work to find balance between sharing and creating space for others. It is important to have the courage to share your thoughts with those around you. But if you find your mind is racing with thoughts, take your time and make space to be exposed to someone else's perspective that may challenge your own ideas, values, and perspectives.

3. Keep an open mind: It's okay to not know everything. The more readily we accept our own ignorance, the more space we create for new understanding.

4. Use "I" statements: Speak from your own experience, not the assumption of others. Conversely, these are not your experiences to judge. This is a gift of vulnerability in action.

5. Name the feeling. We feel all things on our bodies. As you are a part of the discussion, name what comes up for you. Ask yourself, why?

6. Transparent accountability: We have to hold ourselves accountable for both the spaces we are a part of and the spaces we create. What

are we bringing to the space we are in, including ideologies or experiences we are still processing?

7. This is a living document: Learning is constant and our needs change. These agreements that we make with one another may evolve as we are exposed to more bodies, ideas, and feelings. We can make space at any time to build upon them or change something that excludes or limits community.

And, of course, we must not forget that the foundation of this space is love.

In a world that continues to separate us from ourselves internally and the ways that we learn and build with others, it's important that we understand the only strategy that will eradicate oppression is if we are connected. It is in our connection that we find our collective power and are a true threat to those in power. Fitness 4 All Bodies reminds us that this connection framed in love is the only way.

CHAPTER 2

Unknowing the Gym: Moving toward Imagination as Liberation

LAWRENCE KOVAL

During the summer of 2020, I was a graduate student at UNC-Chapel Hill about to enter my second year in a two-year folklore MA program. Most of the United States was still in a state of lockdown due to the exponentially devastating COVID-19 pandemic. As a country, we experienced the first swell of cases and deaths that summer—though that would then be completely overshadowed by the crest in cases that coming winter—and hospitals were and remain today in sore need of beds, staff, and resources.

On May 25, 2020, George Floyd was murdered in Minneapolis, Minnesota, by police officer Derek Chauvin with officers Tou Thao, James Alexander Kueng, and Thomas Kiernan Lane on standby.

Floyd's murder was the proverbial spark on a bed of dry tinder made of the seemingly endless extrajudicial killings and brutality carried out by police officers, especially against Black, Brown, Indigenous, houseless, queer, trans, and disabled people.

The resulting summer was defined by extremes, where the collective grief endured was as deep as the power of collective action. Where we grappled with how to mourn hundreds of thousands of people dying from a novel virus, people showed up by feeding hungry neighbors, demanding support from the government, hand sewing masks, and learning what "mutual aid" meant.

Grief ran deep in mourning the lives stolen by the violence of white supremacy: Breonna Taylor, Ahmaud Arbery, George Floyd, Tony McDade, and so many others. Some people mourned what they thought was a country based in opportunity and freedom rather than genocide, violence, and exploitation. Some mourned the inability to ever believe it was anything but the latter. But where headlines reported "division" and insisting on unity through silence, togetherness and commitment could be found on the streets where hundreds of thousands of people gathered to insist that #BlackLivesMatter.

We are often convinced that historical moments play out like a movie, where we experience almost omniscient clarity about how and when to get involved and that one major moment will always be a greater solution than tiny acts of collectivity and persistence. But if you ask generations of people who have engaged in resistance work, they'll remind you how the headlines we read are borne out of many other everyday moments and all the mundaneness in between.

It looks like putting on sunscreen before going out to protest. It looks like seeing pictures of radicals and revolutionaries riding bikes, enjoying summer, and laughing with their friends and families. It looks like reading a new book just for pleasure or learning how to crochet because it is just as important to remember what joy, contentedness, and calm feel like in a chaotic, activating world.

It is in that in betweenness that the question arises: What about gyms?

It could seem a bit ridiculous to think about gyms when considering revolutionary action, but this sense of irrelevancy or unrelatedness is by design. In general, we are encouraged to leave what are seen as "leisure" or "recreational" activities as completely unexamined.

This is part of what makes them leisurely, you might say, the ability to just engage in them mindlessly. But when we look at how white supremacy is perpetuated, it is in these purposefully unexamined spaces that it is maintained as the status quo most rigidly. When we talk about systems of inequality and inequity, it is systems we are talking about. This means that even if there were no people serving as actors and bringing in their own personal behaviors and biases, these systems would still uphold white supremacy as a structure of power through the patterns they construct, values they uphold, and ideas they naturalize.

Gyms are no exception.

One of the ways the fitness-industrial complex* maintains its power is by convincing people that gyms and fitness spaces are inherently apolitical and exist separate from the rest of our public and private lives. In reality, they are spaces where ideas of body citizenship in a white supremacist system are constructed and played out.

When someone checks in at their local Planet Fitness, they likely aren't asking themselves why certain metrics appear on the dashboard of the treadmill, how gym spaces were developed, or why we are always telling ourselves we constantly need to lose five, ten, fifteen pounds. I'm not saying they should be asking these questions at every encounter, because sometimes we just need to get through our day. But what I'm trying to say is that when we enter gym and fitness spaces there are a thousand incremental elements we completely take for granted and even come to expect, or require, from these spaces.

Imagine a gym. Maybe you started to imagine one when I mentioned Planet Fitness. For a moment, just consider what elements are present there. If you're imagining people, who is using what equipment? Why are people

---

* As defined by Justice Roe Williams.

there? What do they look like? What is the gym, as this space of convergence, trying to accomplish?

Now that we have this image of a bustling, daresay successful gym in our minds, let's take it apart and render it useless. Would removing particular items or machines render it decidedly not a gym? As for the people in the gym, what are their wrong reasons to be there? What makes their time at the gym useless? What are the wrong ways to use the equipment? Think beyond your typical misadventures. Imagine someone using a treadmill as their desk because the gym is their satellite office for the day. Imagine children using the dumbbells as blocks. Someone signing up says they can't wait to be lazy, to gain weight, to look less toned, and to just use the gym as a place to nap and read a book.

You might be thinking, "obviously, gyms are places where people work out and that there's certain expectations for results; that's why a gym is called a gym." And you're completely correct. But what I'm hoping this begins to do is denaturalize the gym, aka dig up all those assumptions and expectations for us to examine, and inspire you to start asking questions about why gyms exist the way they do and for what purpose. For example, why are treadmills, ellipticals, and stationary bikes the cardio machines we see in gyms versus those fun vibrating massagers from spas in the '50s? The answer that popped into your head might be something like because those machines actually work—and it is this idea of "working" and "results" that I want to hold on to for a second.

When people step into fitness spaces like gyms or studios, they often have a goal in mind. Let's stick with this idea of losing weight or getting stronger as those are pretty ubiquitous motivators. Already, there is the idea that the body will be changed and transformed in a particular direction. Namely, toward strength or toward thinness.

"No, shit," you might think. "What's the point otherwise? You think we should run on the treadmill aimlessly and lift weights just because?" I would ask, why not? And why does that seem like an antithesis to what these spaces require? Because if we were to ask someone about their goals and why they want to lose weight or get stronger, we might be met with answers like "It's healthier" or "It'll make me feel better about my body." But if we were to ask again, "Why is it healthier?" or "Why would it make you feel better?"

we might get answers about how it's better to be "fit," ideas of "healthiness," avoiding "laziness," or "just because."

Overall, these ideas reveal that the gym is traditionally a space to make the body a project and specifically one that values thinness, strength, and "healthiness." The implications of this may not yet be clear if this is your first time deconstructing the idea of the gym, but if you are familiar, it is unsurprising especially if we consider the historical origins of the gym in America and its goals.

Physical Culture and Its Development in the United States

To better understand how origin of physical culture and gyms in the United States is at the intersection of eugenics, nationalism, and gender politics, one must understand the dominant culture at the time they were developed. As David Churchill describes, during the late nineteenth century urban city centers were continuing to grow, and increasing numbers of middle-class Americans saw the cities they lived in as immoral, unhealthy places in comparison to the myth of idyllic, pure pastoral living.[1]

In these cities, there were increasingly more "white collar" jobs for the middle class that did not demand the levels of physical exertion that working the land did. As a result, there were growing social anxieties that men—specifically white men—were becoming soft in both body and spirit, and there were growing anxieties over how this would affect the collective national "body."

During this same timeframe, the developing concepts of evolution, heredity, and natural selection were being adopted to fortify nationalist, imperialistic, and thus white supremacist rhetoric. With the publication of Charles Darwin's works *On the Origin of Species* (1859) and *The Descent of Man* (1871), ideas such as "survival of the fittest" and "natural selection" were adopted into this social context to implement the idea of "social Darwinism."

Industrial capitalists used this concept in the late nineteenth century as "an apology for competition and force."[2] Previously, the origins of different racial groups were continuously debated, with those supporting monogeny arguing that all races derived from a single origin, whereas polygeny proponents argued that different races descended from separate biological and geographical sources.[3] With the introduction of evolutionary theory, "the notion of visible differences and racial hierarchies were deployed to corroborate Darwinian theory."[4]

In 1883 Francis Galton coined the term *eugenics* to describe the developing "science" around heredity. Eugenics-based initiatives sought—and perpetuate today in the same vein—to essentially perfect whiteness through phenotypic and performance-based traits:

> The widespread scientific and social interest in eugenics was fueled by anxieties expressed through the popularized notion of (white) "race suicide." This phrase, invoked most famously by Theodore Roosevelt, summed up nativist fears about a perceived decline in reproduction among white Americans. The new field of eugenics worked hand in hand with growing antimiscegenation sentiment and policy, provoked not only by attempts for political representation among African-Americans but also by the influx of large populations of immigrants. As Mark Haller has pointed out, "Racists and [immigration] restrictionists . . . found in eugenics the scientific reassurances they needed that heredity shaped man's personality and that their assumptions rested on biological facts."[5]

"Anthropometry" arose as a means to divide people based on physical differences. This focus on quantifying and measuring the body created the assumption that through the body were "various keys or languages available for reading its logic of biological determinism, the surface and interior body rather than its social characteristics, such has clothing, became the primary sites of meaning."[6]

Dudley Sargent was an American follower of Galton and his anthropometric interests. Sargent was a physical culture enthusiast himself and a Harvard educator whose priority was building the "harmonious body," a body that is symmetrical and proportioned. Where Galton and Sargent schools of thought diverged is that Sargent believed physical and mental abilities could be developed rather than solely being procured by genetics. As a result, "building the harmonious body was something that almost anyone could accomplish, even by individuals who did not have 'natural endowment.'"[7]

As Churchill states, "Physical Culture was a broad term used to describe a range of exercises, athletics, and outdoor activities." Within physical culture, there were two main schools of thought. The first suggested gymnastics, calisthenics, and weight training for strengthening the body and building muscle. This first wave of physical culture held distinctly European origins. During the nineteenth century, the gymnastics movement was alive and well throughout Germany and its separate states. With the significant influx of German immigrants to the United States after the 1848 revolution, immigrant communities would bring with them their forms of physical culture, which many American health and fitness groups eventually integrated into their own programs. The second vision advocated for sports programs such as football with the argument that games and sports taught "comradeship and values." Furthermore, athletics were linked with nationalism and the idea that these games demonstrated the country's democratic spirit. This focus on sports constituted the second wave of programming offered and advocated for, but never truly replaced the first approach to physical culture.[8]

Advocacy for physical culture pre-dates the adoption of exercise rhetoric by eugenicists, given that during the early part of the nineteenth century, "health advocates had encouraged exercise as a way of warding off disease ... early health enthusiasts were not just concerned with healthy bodies ... [but] 'healthy' minds and spirits to go along with one's body."[9] The Young Men's Christian Association (YMCA) was founded in industrial London in 1844 as a refuge to study the Bible and to transcend the regimented class divisions. Inspired by these stories of the YMCA in England, Thomas Valentine Sullivan founded the first YMCA in the United States at the Old South Church in Boston, Massachusetts, on December 29, 1851.[10]

By the late 1880s and early 1890s, YMCAs began to diverge from their more explicitly evangelical purposes to instead invest in gymnastics programming that "sought to build bodies rather than save and uplift souls."[11] As a result, YMCAs employed hundreds of full-time staff members responsible for physical training programs and developing a culture where "training of the body was part of the modern routine of work, leisure, family, and volunteerism, part of the everyday experience of the contemporary and efficient gentleman."[12] During the latter part of the nineteenth century, this intersection of physical health, muscular development, and Christian morality led to the rise of "Muscular Christianity," first popularized in Great Britain and then the United States, which "provided a Protestant response to fears of effeminacy and moral decline."[13]

Of course, the role of muscularity in constructing masculinity has fluctuated and changed over time.[14] While male gym-goers had their sexuality questioned in the 1930s,[15] the emphasis on the male body increased during other time periods such as the 1970s and 1980s, with muscularity becoming a central component of constructing dominant forms of masculinity. Bodybuilding became a space to establish hypermasculinity even with its connections to "hustler" culture—namely, gay sex work.[16] Similarly, "physique magazines" and competitions acted as "discreet avenues for closeted gay men to find each other in intolerant times."[17] Arnold Schwarzenegger was quoted saying, "You will find homosexuals signing up to become members of the group so they can just watch you working out . . . to them we are heaven" and reassuring men that they "shouldn't feel like fags because they want to have nice-looking bodies," using stories about "gang bangs" and casual sex with women, highlighting the ever-present construction of masculinity through both fitness and misogyny.[18] Meanwhile, women were often not allowed to engage in athletic pursuits, and the ones who did were labelled as being hypermasculine.[19] Additionally, women attended beauty parlors of the 1930s–1950s that utilized machines focused on "slenderizing" and thus feminizing the body.

By the 1970s and 1980s, figures such as Jane Fonda and Arnold Schwarzenegger appeared as prominent starlets of these developing lineages of activity focusing on ideas of "wellness," "health," and engaging in a new form of work ethic centered around bodily transformation.[20] For men, it was an emphasis on muscularity, thus developing an exaggerated form of this pursuit through body building.[21] While there were women who were professional bodybuilders during this time, places such as aerobics or yoga studios became "third spaces"* created for women and gay men to congregate within.[22] In particular, scholar Natalia Petrzela highlights the lineages of celebrity aerobics instructor Jane Fonda, Jazzercise founder Judi Sheppard Missett, and Esalen Institute's founding yoga instructor Pamela Rainbear Portugal in mapping these third spaces and creating places and ways where women felt like they could work out publicly and in community.

It is worth making explicit that these studio spaces similarly center whiteness, much like the origin of the gym. Petrzela argues that these spaces and lineages are liberatory in nature, particularly through providing these community spaces and creating new ways for women to be in their bodies— thus pushing back against the frequent critique that wellness and fitness subcultures are inherently based in narcissism. It seems worth stating that both resisting against particular standards and reinscribing aspects of dominant culture—such as whiteness, classism, and so forth—are not mutually exclusive.

This is captured to some extent in Alan Klein's ethnography, *Little Big Men: Bodybuilding Subculture and Gender Construction*, with professional bodybuilders in California during the late '80s and early '90s. Devoting a chapter to female bodybuilders, he captures this gray area created where women have to carve out spaces for themselves in the industry—especially one he identifies as actively utilizing narcissism and fascist bodily aesthetics in their identity construction—while still not being feminists or having any desire to engage in any explicit form of liberation. When one female bodybuilder is asked about entering the sport, she shares that when professional body building was opened to women, it attracted people who wanted to stir things up, "feminists," and other people who were invested in the transgressive nature of the sport. But, she says, those women had left, and the remaining female bodybuilders were actually being devoted to the sport rather than having any interest in making a statement.[23]

---

* Also known as *third place*, this concept is defined by Ray Oldenburg in his book *The Great Good Place* (1989) as being a crucial social space that is separate from the other primary social environments of the home (first place) and work (second place).

While Klein's work primarily focuses on male bodybuilders and the specific form of masculinity they construct—which he terms "comic book masculinity"—this focus on women entering hypermasculine gym spaces dominates the literature of the past few decades in regards to looking at the relationship between gender and the gym. For example, Shelly A. McGrath and Ruth A. Chananie-Hill interviewed female bodybuilders at a midwestern university with particular interest and emphasis on women's gender in relationship to body building. While muscularity is historically and culturally tied to the ideal performance of hegemonic masculinity,[24] these women engaged in a "both/and" means of both transgressing and reaffirming expected gender roles. They transgress gender boundaries by continuing to engage in what are seen as "masculinizing" activities despite these gender regulations while asserting their own femininity, while still reinscribing particular gender norms by demarcating a line at which someone is "like a man," such as using steroids, or continuing to connect "looking like a man" to lesbianism.[25]

This idea that women who are more muscular are lesbians is not a new narrative. The hypermasculinization of women who exercise can be traced from the origins of the gym itself[26] to the 1990s as presented in a scene in Klein's ethnography in California following professional bodybuilders. When a film crew comes in to film a segment about female bodybuilders, a man yells, "Hey, they [women] already got doctors, lawyers, cops, and now bodybuilders! The next thing you know, they'll wanna be queer!"[27]

Quoting bell hooks, "Black women have long been portrayed as masculine and inappropriately feminine in popular media; athletes are popular targets for this negative attention because of their muscles and physical prowess."[28] In "Misogynoir in Medical Media: On Caster Semenya and R. Kelly," Moya Bailey points to the clear examples of Venus and Serena Williams, who are often considered to be "too aggressive and too masculine to compete with other (read: white) competitors" as well as Caster Semenya, a Black intersex woman and Olympic gold medalist, whose name filled the headlines when her status as intersex became a topic of intense speculation.[29] Semenya was subjected to extensive "gender testing" for the sake of confirming that she was "truly a she," from her hormonal levels being tested to her organs being

X-rayed. The invasion of her privacy and global sensationalism resulted in her being placed on suicide watch. As Bailey states, "The specter of the Black woman's body at the intersections of socially constructed and medically reinforced hierarchies of biological difference remains a trope in contemporary media and dates back to our earliest uses of mass communications."[30] Even as advocates for Semenya defended her, they—perhaps unintentionally—reiterate the same anxieties that produced this situation of medical misogynoir and fear of the nonstandard body:

> Another official suggested that Semenya was being depicted as a monster, which was the kind of thing that drives someone to suicide. In the minds of those trying to protect her, affirming Semenya's femininity and womanhood was essential to her humanity, suggesting their own fear of the non-normative body.[31]

Although masculinity and particularly exaggerated forms of it are central to fitness culture, the feminization of the space, culture, and practices does not inherently make it inclusive, given the often-exclusive nature of femininity itself—as demonstrated by the experience of Caster Semenya.

This relationship between whiteness, femininity, and fitness spaces is further emphasized by Maxine Leeds Craig and Rita Liberti's 2007 study focusing on a women-only gym franchise with the pseudonym "GetFit." In seeking to answer whether a women-only gym is truly "femininized"—or rather, questioning whether the dynamics of power are truly changed if only women engage in it—they found that the dynamics are different without men in the space, but it still constructs an exclusive form of femininity—one that centers heterosexuality, cisgender identity (though this is not even brought up as a factor to consider), whiteness, thinness, and affluence. It is worth noting how working class men may be more likely to turn to fitness as a means of engaging with hegemonic masculinity, whereas women often access fitness as a means of indicating higher class status and affluence.

This exclusive form of femininity is produced through the gym emphasizing weight loss as nearly the only available goal for engaging in the space by regularly measuring participants and publicly sharing how many inches women have lost, asking questions such as whether someone was the same weight on their wedding day prior to the Marriage Equality Act being signed into law, and nearly all social small talk being centered around husbands and children. Additionally, white participants would qualify their interview statements describing staff or other clients with racial identifiers and would explicitly talk about modifying the conversations around racially neutral topics—one participant said they maybe would not talk about skiing with a Black gym goer. Other conversations with white participants included talking about the racial makeup of different locations and comparing it with friends.[32]

Fitness culture's exclusivity extends beyond solely individual actions and performances; the gym "does gender."[33] One of the ways that the gym does gender and guides gender performance and enactment is through how the gym is constructed as a "themescape," a place of hyperreality, becoming "hegemonic, mediating the experience of environments beyond themselves."[34] How this manifests is creating a space where men are allowed, and expected, to take on the role of loud, sweating, weight-slamming meatheads, whereas women are expected to silently relegate themselves to the cardio machines, wear outfits specifically made for the gym, make sure not to work too hard, and not expect to be considered experts or have ownership over the space.

The gym also spatially guides gender performance and construction through what equipment is available and how the space is laid out. For example, women are guided toward cardio machines and lighter weights and men toward heavier weights through the layout of the space, such as the location of locker rooms.[35] This was demonstrated at GetFit as well through part of the gym's "feminization" being an explicit rearrangement of equipment. Rowing machines are often lined up side by side and sometimes facing a mirror in a "traditional" gym focused on individual performance, but at GetFit rowing machines were placed in a circle, essentially requiring that users socialize and orient toward one another.[36] Additionally, GetFit utilized a set of stations set in a circular routine that participants are meant to cycle through, similarly requiring cooperation while negating the need to assert oneself to use a machine otherwise required in traditional gyms.[37]

Consider how the gym as a themescape also exaggerates other dimensions of positionality and identity such as class, ability, race, and so forth and the discrepancies that exist between the dominant cultures and identities enshrined in these spaces versus those excluded. Even further, one of the unifying elements of all of this literature is that its true hostility appears in a coded fashion: through body size.

Regardless of if you're performing masculinity or femininity, in the gym, body size is the "common enemy." Writers such as Dr. Sabrina Strings and Da'Shaun L. Harrison have discussed the connection between anti-fatness and anti-Blackness in their books *Fearing the Black Body: The Racial Origins of Fat Phobia* (2019) and *Belly of the Beast: The Politics of Anti-Fatness as Anti-Blackness* (2021), respectively. Fatness has also been described as being inherently queer, gender nonconforming, or prevents individuals from being read as performing gender in the same way as thin/straight-size people are. This applies to reading fatness as queer if we consider queerness as deviating from the norm—where thinness is held at its center—as well as the material realities of how fatness affects gender performance and how gender is read.[38] Demonizing fatness becomes a coded means of reinscribing white supremacist culture through privileging and enshrining the white, cisgendered, heterosexual, thin, non-disabled body while utilizing Western medicine as a means of justifying said hatred and exclusion of fatness through ideas of "health."

This should demonstrate that fitness or gyms are not simply neutral space where anyone can enter and decide to "work out." Rather, gyms and fitness are inscribed with and enact white supremacist cultural ideals through the bodies they emulate and center and who they castigate. Even potential acts of resistance or transgression can be subjugating in attempts to achieve limited "inclusivity" rather than moving toward broader liberation. Additionally, the canonical fatphobia of fitness culture and spaces, under the guise of promoting good health, creates a coded way of engaging in racism, misogyny, homophobia, ableism, and so forth while being able to maintain the image of seemingly being a neutral space where anyone can enter and decide to work out.

The Body Positivity Movement and Co-optation

Even radical movements that have sought to address this disparity have to wrestle with not just fighting a system head-on, but the way white supremacy co-opts and dilutes movements against power structures into the arena of the individual.

The body positivity movement is thought to have originated in the 1960s as a movement demanding the "radical acceptance of marginalized bodies." This included severing the link between health and weight, addressing systemic issues such as fat communities facing employment discrimination and medical prejudice, and understanding the intersectional nature of fatness and other marginalized identities. As Cheryl Frazier and Nadia Mehdi excellently articulate in "Forgetting Fatness: The Violent Co-optation of the Body Positivity Movement,"[39] the body positivity movement was ripped from its roots and violently co-opted by thin people—especially white cisgender women—as well as companies and corporations in an unethical manner that leaves the original harms that the movement sought to address unresolved. Instead, the focal point was forcibly shifted from the systemic issues to instead focus upon ideas of self-love or the idea that body positivity is able to be accomplished on the individual level alone. As the authors acknowledge, things such as self-love and empowerment are not necessarily inherently antithetical to the overall movement. The issue is when these tenets become weaponized to completely replace the initial goals and completely decenter the main population affected, fat people, with thin bodies to create new boundaries around "acceptable fatness."

This bleeds over into fitness, given the way weight and fitness are so deeply enmeshed with one another, where the gym becomes a confessional booth to repent for erring, returning the body to a state of disciplined thinness and hegemonic aesthetic.[40] The body is treated as a moral project where thinness indicates discipline and fatness indicates personal failure—regardless of how this connects to actual effort and setting aside the fact that working out doesn't necessarily translate into body composition.

Unknowing the Gym

I've spoken here about what gyms have historically perpetuated and enacted, but if we return to the idea of "in betweenness," we can catch a glimpse of what gyms could be. During the spring and summer of 2020, many gyms and fitness spaces were closed in America due to state-issued ordinances prohibiting certain businesses from operating in-person, particularly those that posed a higher chance of spreading COVID-19, such as gyms and bars. Paired with the uprisings to support the Black Lives Matter movement, the growing economic crisis mass unemployment, and the upcoming presidential election, the hum and flow of the status quo had ground to a halt. The machine of capitalism was creaking, and headlines talked about collapse. While the most marginalized groups had always been aware of and experienced these shortcomings, they were now affecting white, middle-class families. This shift meant the failures of capitalism—and the white supremacist system of power its fuels—were being put on display and made explicit rather than being able to be hidden in the rhetoric of "pull yourself up by your bootstraps."

But while real suffering and consequences exist for people within those gaps, those spaces of in between also give way to incredible resilience and creativity. This was particularly profound to witness with gyms and fitness spaces during this time. Gyms and studios already exist as a transitory space, but maybe this is what gives them the special kind of potential for creation and change that has been witnessed historically and was showcased during 2020.

Through social media, I was able to watch as gyms in New York City opened their doors as places for protestors to reconvene, charge their phones, get water, and use the bathroom. An initiative known as Town Fridge installed a community fridge outside Radically Fit Oakland. Other places distributed masks, held fundraisers, and invested in mutual aid. Organizations like Fitness 4 All Bodies (F4AB) hosted webinars and workshops discussing the need to go beyond diversity and inclusion in gyms—to acknowledge what gyms are founded upon and create new foundations and roots to grow from.

Many of the people involved in this educational work have spoken about the possibilities of what gyms could be, as community spaces and being explicit about their political nature, for decades. Some have worked under the umbrella of "body positive," but as discussed by Frazier and Mehdi the co-optation around body positivity has required a shift in language to be explicit in its connotations. As a result, a number of activists, fitness professionals, and communities have gravitated toward *inclusive fitness*. Even among those who use this terminology there are some caveats to express, but there is a loose agreement that the utility of the term as a common phrase to indicate what they mean makes it worth using.

I had the privilege of talking to a number of people affiliated with F4AB and part of its larger community—and many who are contributors to this very text—about the concept of inclusive fitness and spaces of possibility, including Justice Williams (Fitness 4 All Bodies), Roc Rochon (Rooted Resistance), Ilya Parker (Decolonizing Fitness), Dr. Joy Cox (Jabbie App), Dr. Courtney Marshall, Asher Freeman (Nonnormative Body Club), Lore McSpadden (Positive Force Movement), and Beck Beverage. Everyone I talked to had been advocating for changes in the industry through their own or other collective endeavors in addition to their work with F4AB.

During our conversations, there were a few specific themes that I focused on:

- What defines "traditional" fitness versus "inclusive" fitness
- What constitutes "exercise" and "fitness"
- Labor conditions within the fitness industry
- Hopes and desires for what fitness could offer and become
- Efforts they've put forward to create the fitness spaces and practices to meet these desires

These discussions contained a wealth of knowledge and experience, including recounting experiences from playing on the playground and what that felt like in their body to learning how to lift weights as an adult. The state of exercise and fitness itself was questioned, such as asking why walking on a treadmill is considered exercise but manual labor like sweeping or beating a rug is not. From these experiences I gathered that "inclusive fitness," or whatever we decide to call it, is ultimately a movement toward unknowing.

Unknowing Carcerality

White supremacy perpetuates itself through carceral systems. Schools become places to surveil and train future workers under racial capitalism. Psych wards and prisons alike hide people, social problems, and suffering within white supremacist society and punish "unruly" bodyminds. Even whiteness, cis-genderedness, heterosexuality, able-bodiedness, neurotypicality—these all operate as panopticons where actual belonging to these discrete categories is conditional, illusory, and ever-shrinking. Instead, we are encouraged to police ourselves and police one another. The scapegoating of anyone at the edges makes the boundaries around their construction increasingly tighter and more rigid. How is the gym—as it's currently conceived and enacted—not a carceral institution itself where we are encouraged to make good "body citizens" out of ourselves along these same lines?

Much like prisons are presented as singular, punitive solutions to expansive, multifaceted social issues, how is the pursuit of a singular standard of "health," such as by way of weight loss, or the canonized body (white, thin, abled, etc.), not the equivalent singular solution to various issues, needs, and experiences of diverse bodies? Thus, it is not undue to suggest that abolition is a lens through which we can consider gyms and fitness, as well.

Abolition extends beyond the dissolution or especially the reinvention of prisons, or simply creating another singular solution just by another name; it erodes at the idea of these solutions and even questions the nature of "solution" in the first place.[41] Abolition is stepping away from certainty, absolute knowing, and prescriptive answers. As Liat Ben-Moshe suggests in *Decarcerating Disability: Deinstitutionalization and Prison Abolition* (2020), abolition need not promise that things inherently get better, either. In doing so, it would actually preclude its own abilities. Promising that abolition is its own solution threatens to inculcate it into the same system it seeks to fight. Rather, we can only know that the current system we operate within is dehumanizing and needs to be torn apart. Given the way our preexisting knowledge of people, society, and relationships is so deeply defined by carceral systems, we likely cannot even begin to imagine what we can do going forward until its very dissolution. We will likely need to reinvent again and again.

While the systems threatened by abolition like to frame it as only destructive, maligning, and divisive, ultimately it is this imagination that it centers around. To quote Alexis Pauline Gumbs—scholar, poet, activist, writer based in the city I write this now, Durham, North Carolina:

> What if abolition is something that sprouts out of the wet places in our eyes, the broken places in our skin, the waiting places in our palms . . . what if abolition is something that grows?[42]

It is this move toward unknowing and creation that was present in my conversations with everyone I talked to. They questioned what constitutes "exercise" and "fitness" in the first place, wanting to leave that for people themselves to decide what determines those categories. They pushed back against the idea of prescriptive workouts or one-size-fits-all programming, instead centering people, their experience, and own bodily knowledge to take the precedent when it comes to guiding any sort of movement practice. We discussed moving without a specific goal or purpose, moving for pleasure, and moving just to be in the company of other people we care about. Rather than centering answers, our conversations sought out questions when it comes to fitness practices and spaces.

That also invited contradiction, such as competing access needs, a concept from disability rights where someone's access needs may be at odds with someone else's. Or being trans and wanting to work out to achieve a specific aesthetic to be able to pass, while recognizing the inherent issues that come with that. Or recognizing that trying to lose weight may be something someone needs to do to exist in a deeply fatphobic society.

These conversations exist in those gaps that became more visible over the course of these past few years, just like is the case with any wide-reaching historical event. And not only do they exist within the gaps, these questions and conversations seek to expand that space until the only space we have left is to simply be without restriction and to determine what boundaries we want to set for support rather than constriction.

Return to the image of the gym that you built up and broke down. Does entering the gym without a goal in mind truly break the gym, or simply change it? What's wrong with someone sleeping on the treadmill or a bench if that's where they're safe? What requires breaking in order to build something new? How do we build spaces and practices that preserve and protect our humanity? How can we create more space for ourselves and for other people?

CHAPTER 3

My Body, My Anarchy

M CAMELLIA

I touch my own skin, and it tells me that before there was any harm, there was miracle.

—adrienne maree brown

This year, for the first time in my adult life, I started taking care of my skin. Maybe it was the onset of my thirties, or reflecting on my mom's recent brush with skin cancer. Maybe it was the harshness of winter on my face, the flush I couldn't seem to cool, the sensitivity I couldn't bear. It could have been the strong anti-authoritarian impulse in me reacting to the oft-repeated pandemic-era instruction not to touch my face. Or, perhaps more likely, it might have been the pandemic-era isolation in all of its manifestations—the single-weekend binge watch of *Queer Eye*, the seemingly unending desire to be touched, and the recurrent, urgent tug of my tanking dopamine levels compelling me to seek out new forms of pleasure, especially those that didn't require exposure to viral risk or inebriation. Maybe I semiconsciously decided to trade in bottles of wine for bottles of toner and fancy face oil.

The first and only other time I had a skin care routine, it was initiated and overseen by my mother, who rushed me to the Clinique counter in the nearest suburban mall at the first hint of acne, fearing that my face would end up scarred like my father's. As a kid, it would seem, my body and mind were in agreement about wanting to run head-first into adulthood—at eight, I was bullied into shaving my body hair, at nine, surprised by a three-week period, and at ten, prescribed birth control when it never regulated on its own. That same year, I got my first true zit, suddenly filled out a bra, and started to perpetually suck in my stomach after first hearing my doctor say that I weighed more than average for my age. My first serious bout of depression came the year after that.

It was only recently that I realized the common thread of isolation among the other parallels between these two forays into skin care. When I was younger, I would go to bed, squeeze my eyes shut, and play the same reel over and over in my head, hoping to keep out the intrusive thoughts and fears that kept me from falling asleep at night and from getting out of bed in the morning. In that forced vision, I was always grown, always thin and feminine, always standing in a clearing in the woods with an ambiguous man (always a man), taking traditional marriage vows while surrounded by my friends and family, all of them beaming at me, adoring and proud. That imaginary version of myself was, of course, always glowing and euphoric. After all, she was beautiful, beloved, chosen. She belonged.*

In reality, I did have friends and a family, including married parents, then a budding rarity, as well as two younger siblings. I rarely had to be alone, though sometimes I chose to be, especially on the days when I was feeling the least able to connect with the people around me. I often experienced this as overwhelming annoyance that no one in my life seemed to want to talk about the things that I did, usually followed shortly thereafter with the

---

* I use the pronoun "she" here with intention. I am an agender non-binary person who was assigned female at birth, and my pronouns are exclusively they/them/ theirs. However, ten-year-old me didn't have this language and could never even have imagined a reality where the gender binary, its conflation with external genitalia, and default heterosexuality weren't givens. Thus, these imaginary versions of me were always cisgender, heterosexual women.

jump-scare of a thought that I was somehow irreconcilably different, somehow wrong, somehow broken, and that I would never feel happy, secure, or chosen in my truth.

I'm not going to pretend that these intrusive thoughts have stopped completely. Here I am, twenty years later, still reckoning with the occasional onset of that familiar foreboding feeling, that same creeping sense of loneliness and disconnect, sometimes even in the company of my dearest beloveds. It still scares me shitless, at times so much so that when I am lying awake in bed at night with my cats and my insomnia, I'll squeeze my eyes shut and imagine a different reality, yet another future vision with the same themes—beauty, love, pleasure, choice, belonging. Home. Family.

Practicing Pleasure

And. But.

A lot has changed in twenty years. For one, when I stand in front of my bathroom mirror cleansing, toning, exfoliating, moisturizing, putting on my daily SPF in the morning, or oiling it all off at the end of the day, I know that I'm doing it of my own volition, for my own immediate pleasure and long-term benefit. When I touch my skin, it's out of reverence, not enforced shame over my blemishes, nor fear of the very fine wrinkles around my eyes, which will likely deepen with time. I think they've shown up to remind me of the rings inside a tree's trunk, to tell me that I'm a part of nature, part of the cyclical continuum of existence. When I comb out my hair, I no longer hear my mom's voice threatening to cut it off if I don't keep it detangled—I just enjoy the way it feels, its soft strength. I call my grays "tinsel" and enjoy being adorned.

For another, I don't own a scale anymore. I finally inhaled, taking deep breaths fifteen years after first sucking in my stomach, afraid that breathing into my lower lungs made my belly look larger. I wear clothes that fit—sometimes I even design, make, and/or tailor them myself. I hike in Shenandoah and kickbox to Beyoncé in my living room when my body allows because I enjoy feeling strong and feeling the intensity of my breath. I choose to go to therapy, even when things are relatively good, because there will always be more to work through. I'm honest with my psychiatrist and might finally even be on the right mix of medications for my neurochemistry. I still have trouble getting to sleep, but I do get out of bed in the morning.

Also, I know my own pronouns now and love the way they taste in my mouth. They. Them. I know which sensations in my body mean "I want to fuck you" and which ones mean "I aspire to be like you." I know my own propensity to wander blissfully along neurodivergent tangents when I'm giving a lecture or telling a story, know that I have as much capacity for pleasure as I do for pain, and know that there are as many definitions of "family" and "beloved" as there are families and beloveds. I learned how to say no, then yes, then maybe, with confidence. I found a non-abusive relationship with the divine, one which inherently includes a deep and compassionate relationship with myself and a new way of conceptualizing my relationships with others and with the world around me.

When I squeeze my eyes shut and imagine the future, I'm no longer imagining a self that doesn't exist. I'm imagining the self that I am right now—my whole, divine, fat, queer, non-binary, neurodivergent, chronically ill, disabled, soft, strong, miraculous-ass self—in one of infinite satisfying scenarios. I'm purposefully trying to reimagine what is possible in my quest to align my life with my values, and I attempt to allow that vision to shift at the pace of change, rather than spinning static fairy tales that were, ultimately, written by someone else. I'm creating, drafting my future, and doing my best to let that guide my everyday actions and contribute to the co-creation of a more liberated world.

As I've learned to feel my inner "no," it's opened up the opportunity for my inner "yes" to be sought, a lesson in duality that has deeply served me, and which is, in large part, the basis of my current, independent work. Since 2016 I've been working at the intersection of yoga, consent education, and social justice. My offerings, which take many forms, are all heavily informed by yoga philosophy, my personal practice, a background working in movements for sociopolitical change, and the radical work of the Black, intersectional feminist lineage that includes the work of Audre Lorde, bell hooks, adrienne maree brown, Prentis Hemphill, Alexis Pauline Gumbs, and countless others. Each of these thought-leaders has substantially contributed to a de-vilified pleasure politic, particularly for Black and Indigenous people of color, women and femmes, queer and trans folks, and others facing systemic oppression. They have also continued to model the necessary integration of somatics—of bodymind integration and the exploration of inner landscapes—in the work of healing the communal trauma wrought by systemic oppression. Yogis, practicing in the traditions born in the Indus Valley and throughout South Asia, have likewise been modeling this truth for thousands of years, despite how their liberatory spiritual practices have been appropriated by our white supremacist culture, including the fitness and diet industrial complexes, which themselves stem from the taproot of racialized colonization.

I've come to see pleasure as a sort of litmus test for gauging desire, and desire as the primary driver of the will. As stated in the Bṛhadāraṇyaka Upaniṣad, in an early doctrine on karma, a spiritual principle of cause and effect:

Now as a man is like this or like that,

according as he acts and according as he behaves, so will he be;

a man of good acts will become good, a man of bad acts, bad;

he became pure by pure deeds, bad by bad deeds;

And here they say that a person consists of desires,

and as is his desire, so is his will;

and as is his will, so is his deed;

and whatever deed he does, that he will reap.

I've also come to understand that each of us has many layers of desire, which may not always align, if they're even consciously accessible to us. And of course, when we move beyond the individual and into matters of relationship, we certainly encounter misaligned desires between beings. This is true whether we're looking at a single, intimate relationship between two people, or scaling up to look at some of the more complex systems of relationship we construct or impact, such as our communities, countries, cultures, and ecosystems.

Within every relationship, regardless of scale, there is an existent power dynamic, a schema for where power is distributed and how it flows between various bodies. I don't believe we can really understand relationships (let alone how to be in liberated and equitable relationships) without starting from a fundamental understanding of power, the many forms it takes, how and where it's being distributed, and how it is being exchanged, which may or may not be consensual. This is precisely what has led me to the paradigm of consent and agency that I do my best to live by and share with others through my work.

All of this is to say that the ultimate difference between ten-year-old me washing my face and envisioning the future and thirty-year-old me doing the same is access to my own innate power and agency. It's a difference in orientation, in where I'm focusing my internal gaze—with time, self-study, somatic integration, and many, many attempts to bolster my mental health through a wide variety of means, each of which taught me something new. I've turned away from external authorities that seek to wield power over me and my actions, and I've started answering to my own, deep, cellular-level "yes" in as many instances as possible.

Unfortunately, it's not always possible—there are still many, many ways that our dominant culture seeks to keep me, as well as everyone else who holds an oppressed identity, from enacting my own will. Systems of oppression disproportionately grant resource access to those who hold specific, privileged identities, and the rest of us are cut us off from as many basic human pleasures as possible, including liberated sexuality, joyful movement, delicious and nourishing foods in the proper quantities to actually sustain us, and—in whatever ways it can, for as long as it can—self-love and true community care. The fitness-industrial complex and contemporary diet culture are two of the many tools that dominant culture uses to exact control—of our time, our money, our bodies, and our self-image—and keep us from experiencing the pleasure that our own bodies are capable of. The pleasure that could, in turn, help us come to understand what we want and what we need. That could motivate us to act differently. That could turn us into the sort of empowered beings who threaten to dismantle the white supremacist, capitalist status quo.

Empowerment is not accomplished by taking whatever we're given by those who seek to hoard and control power, which I would also term "resources." (Here, I mean the broadest possible definition of the word: time, wisdom, money, social capital, status, platform, physical/emotional/mental energy, and more could all be considered resources.) Empowerment is not accomplished when we are taught as children that our truths are limited by a gender binary, a colonized beauty standard, or rules about who and how to love. It is not accomplished when we model every structure in our society into recursive hierarchies and expect those with less proximity to power and privilege to answer to those who've been arbitrarily assigned more. It's not accomplished in a rape culture, nor in any other culture that seeks to terrorize and coerce us into docility.

Rooted in Constructs

What would my early life have looked like if I'd been raised in a culture that valued my body, my experiences, my existence? What would yours have been like if we lived in a culture that taught you how to feel and define your own deep, cellular-level "yes"? If you, and I, and all of our siblings had been born into a world that wanted us all to thrive equitably, interdependently, and in alignment with the truth of ourselves?

I can't face the reality we live in and not feel heartbreak. I don't think that will change in this lifetime, but it doesn't need to become an identity in and of itself—it can remain a feeling, temporal, if caustic. In fact, I think grief can be a catalyst. It's beyond time to invest in ourselves and in our relationships in ways that facilitate greater agency so that we each may choose which direction we want to face when our grief is ignited. Then, when we're each ready, we can light one another up.

It took me nearly three decades to realize that my body is smarter than my mind alone will ever be, and even longer to realize that these two aspects of myself are not separate. Our brains are as much made of organic flesh and chemicals as any other part of our physical beings. The distinctions we make are wholly a construct, arbitrary divisions, much like the constructs humanity has created to divide people.

Race, gender, and fatness are three such constructs, each built from the branches of the same felled tree. European colonizers, seeking to build and maintain superior socioeconomic power and to claim land and other resources from Indigenous communities, needed ways to justify their actions.

Whiteness, as a concept and identity, was created to alleviate the European cognitive dissonance associated with European violence.* You cannot claim superiority without a hierarchy, and you can't create a hierarchy with only one of anything—you can't stack papers until you pulverize and reconstitute the tree into individual sheets. Likewise, no one group of humans can claim top status without somehow defining the boundaries of their closed group, so just as we have arbitrarily separated mind and body, those looking for power outside of themselves must necessarily sever themselves from the whole.

The gender binary as we are generally taught to understand it was largely defined and made rigid to uphold the construct of whiteness, while also doubling to bolster systemic patriarchy. Gender essentialism is the (socially and scientifically discredited) idea that one's gender and corresponding expression of feminine or masculine traits are defined by some (also discredited notion of) fixed, biological sex. Enforcing a binary based in gender essentialism, and thereby constructing rules for a strict divide between feminine and masculine behavior and gender expression, created not only the possibility of men's superiority, but also fodder for the claim that Black and Indigenous people of color were subhuman. Cultural practices and ways of understanding gender throughout much of the world went against the new European definition of "humanity," which required adherence to the constructed, essentialist gender binary. Unsurprisingly, this is not only a taproot of racism and patriarchy, but also of transphobia and homophobia. (I recommend the work of Alok Vaid-Menon as a source for further learning about the racist and colonialist origins of the gender binary.)

Similar to the construction of gender, the demonization of fatness was also created to further differentiate Europeans, particularly European women and their descendants in the American colonies, from enslaved Africans during the transatlantic slave trade. As Dr. Sabrina Strings, an associate

---

* I recognize that a single paragraph cannot possibly offer any semblance of a complete explanation of this concept. To really do the topic justice, I highly recommend looking into the depth of scholarship that exists around whiteness as a construct, such as the work of W. E. B. Du Bois, James Baldwin, and Ta-Nehisi Coates, and their many contemporaries.

professor of sociology at UC Irvine and author of *Fearing the Black Body: The Racial Origins of Fat Phobia*, summarized in an interview for the University of California's news blog:

> At the onset of the trans-Atlantic slave trade, skin color was often used to determine racial belonging. But by the 18th century, skin color (after years of interracial sex in the colonies) proved a poor sorting mechanism. What we had by the 19th century was a new racial discourse that suggested black people were also inherently voracious. Combine this with the displacement of poor Europeans in the 19th century (i.e., Irish, Southern Italians and Russian Jews), and white Americans were being advised to fear black people, as well as these "degraded" or supposedly "part-black" Europeans, who were also purportedly identifiable by their weight and skin color.[1]

By weaponizing a religious ethic of temperance alongside the burgeoning dominance of white supremacist and patriarchal beliefs and capitalist notions of class, thinness was constructed as the new bodily ideal, achievable by the white, "cultured," Protestant faithful. The same idea of inherent "voracity" among people of color, pitted against white temperance—restraint from pleasure—is significantly, perhaps primarily, responsible for the demonization of desire that Lorde wrote about in "Uses of the Erotic," and which I have also come to understand as a means of abuse, control, and disempowerment that has perpetuated to this day. To Lorde, the erotic is not something relegated to the realm of sexuality alone. It is more broadly applied to any deep, sensual pleasure and present-moment experience that informs the experiencer of their capacity for joy in all areas of life:

> The erotic is a measure between the beginnings of our sense of self and the chaos of our strongest feelings. It is an internal sense of satisfaction to which, once we have experienced it, we know we can aspire. For having experienced the fullness of this depth of feeling and recognizing its power, in honor and self-respect we can require no less of ourselves.[2]

Our bodies have always been powerful, which lends them to being politicized. Each time we've created a hierarchy of bodies and identities, we've added a new aspect to the complex societal power dynamic. And while power dynamics are not inherently inequitable, they are certainly nuanced, intersectional, and opportunities for exploitation if unrecognized or intentionally manipulated. To me, this means that where we hold disproportionate power, we also hold disproportionate responsibility, both to ourselves and to everyone we're in relationship with. It also lends credence to everything we know about somatics, epigenetics, cellular memory, and the informative capacity of movement practices, including asanas, the physical postures or "poses" of yoga.

Unlearning Oppressive Pedagogy

Asana practice, also known as "postural yoga," is only one sliver of a much larger system of spiritual, embodied practice. However, due to its physical nature and external visibility (distinct from the powerful, internal practices that are far more subtle), it has come to dominate the largely appropriated, Westernized practice of yoga to the point that a majority of the world believes that postural yoga constitutes the practice in its entirety, often pitched fallaciously as a workout.

As such, contemporary yoga teachers, myself included, are taught to facilitate asana-only practices that are modeled after fitness classes. And as noted earlier, the fitness-industrial complex's obsession with weight loss, "body sculpting," and assimilation to the body ideals of whiteness are rooted in systemic oppression. What's more, the yoga and fitness industries have been built within the larger dominant culture, absorbing many of its toxic paradigms, including supremacy and hierarchy. In our dominant culture, most of our institutions and systems, from government to education to the nuclear family to workplace organizational charts and beyond, are organized into the same severed and hierarchical power structures as our broader society. Most of us are taught throughout our lives to answer to external authority figures, and we have this reinforced in nearly every space we enter, including the public domain within our police state and carceral system.

As children, most of us attend school in an environment where we're expected to respect an adult teacher who we are told is the keeper of the knowledge (a form of power) we need to survive and succeed, as well as an authority over our bodies and conduct. The message we're sent is clear: the teacher (or the police, your boss, the president, your doctors, those with status such as celebrities, or anyone with more proximity to societal power) has what you need, and therefore, you must obey the teacher in order to obtain the resources they keep. At work, you must obey your boss in order to get paid what you need to survive. In the public domain, you must obey the laws determined by the government and enforced by police, regardless of whether they're just or justly enforced, or else risk your freedom, or even your life itself.

When it comes to yoga or fitness classes, the dynamic is mirrored once again. There is a teacher or instructor, who generally stands at the head of the classroom. This teacher is considered the keeper of knowledge, whether that be knowledge of how to "optimize" your body, keep it safe, or something more esoteric, such as the profound spiritual teachings of a wisdom tradition. Regardless, this person is offered authority by virtue of the power they're imbued with. They tell students what to do with their bodies, and students are expected, whether it's spoken or not, to obey in order to gain access to the resource they came in seeking.

For a variety of reasons this dynamic is problematic, but for our purposes, I'm choosing to focus on the ways in which this mirroring of hierarchical paradigms and disproportionate power distributions serve to reinforce the internalizations we receive from all the other structures we are made to exist within—white supremacy, capitalism, and all their smaller-scale iterations within our relationships and institutions. How could we ever build a just and equitable world, free of these oppressive constructs, unless each and every one of us has the opportunity to access the truth of ourselves? To self-realize and exact agency? How can we recognize our own innate power and bring it forth into the world to create change if we are never offered an opportunity to tap into and realize that power? Realize our own needs, desires, and erotic self-knowledge?

I don't think we can. And this is precisely why the dominant culture seeks to maintain the status quo, in which appealing to external authority is often the only viable option, particularly for the folks most harmed by it. It's as Lorde said: "[The erotic] is an *internal* sense of satisfaction . . . recognizing its power, in honor and self-respect, we can require *no less* of ourselves." (Emphasis mine.) Dominant culture knows the status quo is endangered when the oppressed are able to partake in the pleasures of joyful, self-directed movement, consensual sex with our choice of partners (or consensual withdrawal from a culture of sexuality and reproduction), delicious and nourishing food, clean and ample water—when we know these pleasures, we start to demand them, start to takes steps toward access for all. When we know the pleasure of agency and liberation, even if we've only had the smallest taste of that freedom, we know that nothing less is acceptable.

Our bodies and minds are not separate, and our bodies are smarter than our minds alone will ever be. If we think that spoken or signed or written language is all there is, we are making a grave error and cutting ourselves off from our innate wisdom. My bodymind speaks the language of sensation.* There are many ways of knowing, many dialects of sensation that our bodies use to make their powerful wisdom known to our conscious minds, if we are able to listen and translate. Trauma and oppression cut us off from sensation. An externalized authority orientation renders us inattentive to our own internal dialogue. We miss out on the vast store of power contained within us, and thus the opportunity to use that power in alignment with our own true needs and desires, if we are always answering to someone outside of ourselves.

Consent is at the core of liberation from dominant culture, as it helps us find and assert true agency in our bodies. When I offer workshops on consent, I tell participants that consent is always: (1) clear, (2) coherent, (3) given willingly, and (4) ongoing/revocable. Each tenet is important, but I've spent the most time contemplating and exploring the third. How can any of us know our own will without an internal orientation? How can we clarify for ourselves what we need or desire, let alone make those things known or demand them of the world, without a means of discerning our innate truth from our oppressive internalizations?

It is utter rebellion to practice embodiment in a culture that seeks to sever us from our own will. Our bodyminds are microcosms of truth—beneath our consciousness, they continue to behave in alignment with nature, which is

---

* As one beloved who read this draft for me commented, "*This is a spell.*"

both divine and scientific, two terms that I consider synonymous. If sensation is the language of the bodymind, then intentional movement is one way of conversing, an opportunity to learn the truth of the power we all innately contain. If pleasure is a litmus test of desire, then it's vital that we seek the deepest pleasure we possibly can, the spiritually erotic, and align ourselves as closely as possible with our deepest known desires, allowing them to drive our individual will.

If I can learn to listen to the sensations in my body, and if I can start to author the translational dictionary between my body and my conscious understanding, then an internal dialogue can truly begin, a bidirectional conversation between skin and memory. My indiscernible pieces have so much to remind one another, which is, ultimately, just a remembering of themselves. Of myself. This is also true of the bodies we create between ourselves—the relationships, the communities, the organizations, the nations, and others—in the faux stillness that gives the appearance of relief between my end and your beginning, never truly there, but transformed by our mutual attention, intention, investment, relating. Our communal bodies.

Embodiment in Anarchy

We are interdependent and inextricably connected to one another. What we do impacts the people around us. As we scale up to the realm of more and more complex relationships, what does it look like to orient to the internal landscape of a communal body? I posit that it looks like building a culture of mutuality and consent, one which preserves as much individual sovereignty as possible without allowing any individual will to supersede anyone else's. This inherently requires collaboration and negotiation, skillful communication with one another, as well as knowledge of what we actually want. It also requires the availability of options, the knowledge that those options exist, and the freedom to pursue them. A true "yes" can have no meaning unless a real, viable, and accessible option of "no" also exists. From there, we could add any number of "maybes," which to me are incantations of infinite possibility.

A forced or coerced "yes"—a "yes" given under threat, manipulation, or an exploited power dynamic—is not consent. Withholding information or available options is a form of manipulation. The exploitative, hierarchical power paradigm that creates barriers to material necessities and perpetually inflicts trauma and violence upon oppressed communities presents a constant threat, negating our ability to consent in so many arenas by rendering our "yes" meaningless and our "no" unviable or unconscionably risky. What's more, when we are denied access to forums in which to practice deep self-exploration and choice-making—or when the forums where this could be practiced, such as the spaces that exist for intentional movement and embodiment practice, instead just mirror the dominant paradigm—we end up upholding and even serving the oppressive systems, literally working to embody the will of other people by following commands that may or may not actually serve us our infinitely diverse bodies.

I have been the person taking back-to-back power yoga classes as a way of punishing or completely tuning out of my body, forcing my own dissociation because, as a trauma survivor and oppressed person living in the culture I do, most of what I've known has been domination of my body and restriction of my freedom. But my body is an anarchist. It is anarchy itself. It knows what it needs, what it loves, what it longs for, and it doesn't answer to external authority. Instead, it speaks to me, begs me to be its advocate rather than its adversary, reminds me that we are not separate. We are whole, and our nature is sovereignty.

I offer you the following questions as entry points into yourself. They are questions I have asked myself, and continue to ask myself every day. They are also questions I pose to my beloveds and to those who come to practice yoga with me. I encourage you to pair them with equal parts movement and stillness, in whatever ways your body enjoys. They are:

When you exercise, practice yoga, eat a given meal, have sex, or do anything else with your body, where does your motivation come from? Where does your "yes" come from?

Who is directing what is done with your body, your time, your power? Is it another person—a teacher, an instructor, a partner, a political party? A doctor? Someone with preconceived or misinformed notions of what your body should be? A legacy of racist health science and fatphobia?

A lingering memory of a caretaker standing over your shoulder to make sure you washed your face? Your own scalp's recollection of the comb frantically ripping through, pulling out the hair you were detangling under the threat of severance?

If you take yoga or fitness classes with an instructor, do their instructions offer spaciousness for self-exploration and honoring your own body-mind's needs? If you instruct, are you creating the metaphorical silence necessary for your students to learn from their own bodies, the true teachers in the room?

When you say yes to something, is it because you have a sense that it's something you're supposed to do, based on external sources of authority or internalizations from dominant culture? Do you feel like there are other, equally viable options? Do you know that there is potential for as many viable options as there are people born to this Earth, if only we could all recognize and respect one another's profound power?

Do you know what you want? What you hunger for? What your body-mind responds joyfully to? What will satisfy and satiate you in this life? The shapes your pleasure takes? How and where can you explore your own deepest, atomic-level "yes"? Could you explore it in every moment, every movement, every bite? What would that life look like?

How and where can you create and safeguard opportunities for your beloveds and communities to do the same? Where you hold disproportionate power, how can you use it to clear the barriers that keep others from accessing their own? How can you contribute to building a culture of consent, mutuality, and liberation on every scale?

Have you remembered yet that you are nature, anarchy, and divinity? That you can start a macro-scale revolution within the micro of yourself? That we can demand no less of ourselves than to embody our miracle, which is our birthright, instead of whatever harm we have experienced in this lifetime and the lifetimes of our ancestors?

When you touch your own skin, do you hear it singing to you? Are you dancing your response?

PART II

Personal Experiences with Others and Institutions

CHAPTER 4

Push-Ups and Privilege

JOHN R. BRIDGER

I am just a kid from the Kuskokwim River, raised about three hundred miles away from the nearest road system, city, or commercial gym. What rural Alaska lacks in access to sports, it makes up for in passion for basketball. No football, no baseball, no soccer, but basketball. Basketball is religion in the bush. I learned at a young age that being good at basketball equaled being loved. Playing basketball came easier to me than social skills, easier than kindness, than humility, than accountability, and far easier than being authentically me. So with my baggy basketball shorts scrunched up under my blue jeans, I spent every spare moment trying to sneak off to the court. In the rain, in the snow, the twenty minutes during school lunch, and the fifteen minutes before class would start, you could find me investing. And I was rewarded. I know now that through an unspoken agreement I was trading the chance to be all of me for the shallow love promised to those chasing the idea of "the athlete."

In exchange for a team of brothers, my family's pride, and popularity at school, I internalized and embodied a laundry list of toxic and oppressive beliefs that I continue to try and unpack and unlearn today. I replaced tears, tenderness, gentleness, and compassion with competitiveness, dominance, pseudo-stoicism, and the pursuit of external validation. Instead of confronting my loneliness and the deep emotions I was holding, basketball gave me the option of having a community where the only vulnerability expected was physical. Pushing and risking my body was an easy choice compared to exposing my heart. This turned out to be a recipe for a hurting soul with thick muscles, a bitter tongue, and thin skin. My relationships were just good enough to be effective on the court and shallow everywhere else. My self-judgment, insecurity, and denial lashed out regularly, and even those who were kind to me were pushed away. This fast-paced escape served for about a decade as the fresh coat of paint I would brush on top of the growing rust that was my inner world. Reflecting back on this time in my life, it feels so obvious that I was unhappy, but in the moment I did not know any better and likely would not have been able to identify an issue.

I grew up as a guest and settler in the Yup'ik hub town of Bethel, Alaska. I am eternally grateful for a childhood immersed in a rich Indigenous community surrounded by Elders. My first understanding of culture was grounded in collectivist values, living in relationship with the land, and building a better world for the generations yet to come. My hometown and the Yup'ik people are no strangers to colonization and historical trauma. Yet trauma decontextualized and unhealed often kills. The deaths of far too many childhood friends to substance abuse and suicide left deep wounds in my heart. I have been grieving, healing, and searching for understanding ever since. The love and the grief from my childhood propelled me to seek out my current career as trauma therapist and community psychologist.

I have grown weary of having two faces. My therapist self speaks without hesitation about the history and systems of oppression ever large today in the mental health industry. In the last decade, I have been blessed with mentors and peers who have taught me, humbled me, and continue to foster accountability toward dismantling and decolonizing these systems. I still make many mistakes, and through it all, I feel loved, challenged, and authentic within my community of healers and educators. Teleport us to the gym and you can meet another me. I may have shed the most obvious toxic bravado and commentary of my youth, but I am far from embodying many of the core values so readily visible in my therapist self. I am even further from being an agent of change, a leader, or actively resisting the status quo that makes the fitness industry and most fitness spaces inaccessible and hostile to so many.

As an emerging therapist in my midtwenties I hid my athlete identity from most. Most traits I could imagine being associated with that part of me were bound up with shame. I was motivated to distance myself from labels such as the "jock," the "gym-bro," and all the other patriarchal manifestations of masculinity that currently dominate Western fitness culture. I had met no models of authentic masculinity that reflected who I wanted to be or how I felt. It may be more honest to say that I never even considered looking for these models. So I compartmentalized myself into fragmented parts.

In graduate school I found a community of men who for the first time in my life invited and embodied tenderness, sensitivity, kindness, emotional expressiveness, and authenticity in resistance of the patriarchy. I began to unravel and shed many of the layers of what I thought were necessary components of being "a man." I learned to cry again, to listen, to communicate collaboratively, and to begin opening a well-guarded heart. Yet in the midst of finding myself, I could not yet imagine how the athlete would be in harmony with this new me. Instead, for the first time since childhood, I completely stopped going to the gym. I needed to prove to myself that I could be loved for my heart and not just for my athletic abilities.

When I did return to the gym, you could find me with my hoodie up, my headphones on, and all my favorite personality traits left in the car outside the 24-Hour Fitness. I played pick-up basketball for the last time in 2017 after another player attempted to fight me and I watched the ghosts of my old toxic self arise. The hot anger, the ego, the masquerade as a tough guy with my chest puffed out and my forehead pressed against his. A cascade of thoughts and feelings that I no longer recognized as part of me and no longer valued in others or myself. Ironically, this behavior often is effective in gaining the respect of other men, or at least other men who have similarly restricted expressions of masculinity. After heads had cooled and the game was over, I put my basketball shoes into storage and have not played since.

My fitness story is still a rough draft. I am thirty-one years old and have fallen in love with weight lifting. I love the process, the deliberate practice of technique, the ever-growing awareness of my body, and the empowering development of trust in both my physical and mental strength. I enjoy the flexible routine, the growing moments of connection and community, and the privilege of having a reliable space to channel the kinetic overload of energy that builds in me each day.

While I may be in love with weight lifting, my relationship with weight lifting culture could be better described as shamefully codependent. The itchy irony of the commercial gym for me is that I can disappear into myself while every norm around me betrays my values. As a tall, physically strong, white, straight, able-bodied, cis man, I have rarely ever been questioned or messed with in gyms. Aside from the occasional direct compliments I receive, I have the comfortable invisibility of being accepted in a space that has been built aggressively for, and by, people who look just like me.

Highlighting my privilege even further, I believe there are very few things I would be restricted from doing in most fitness spaces. The risks taken for wearing certain clothing, initiating challenging conversations, or directly defying fitness norms are risks to my comfort, not dangers to my personal or physical safety. Given the grace afforded to white cis men, I am actually more likely to be celebrated as a "good man" for things with as low of bar as not hitting on women, not bullying others, and being considerate of the space I am sharing. This is only slightly less problematic than the ways I would be rewarded if I were to embrace the toxic masculinity dripping from most weight rooms.

So how do I end up writing a chapter in this book today? About three years ago I started to intentionally address this incongruence in myself. I began to question what it meant to be consistently and transparently accountable across the spaces in my life. I began seeking others to explore masculinity with, to learn revolutionary approaches to creating fitness spaces, and to work toward finding harmony in myself.

I transitioned to a small barbell club where I could attempt to build community and begin to have the conversations I believe needed to be had. I started stumbling into opportunities that I was underqualified for and was grateful for all the same. I have had the chance to host talking circles between powerlifters on vulnerability, racism, and mental health, to write about my experiences, and to co-facilitate a discussion group that brings together cis and trans men to unpack and reframe masculinity.

When I started asking questions, searching for trainings online, and following new accounts on social media, I quickly learned that I am far from alone in my desire for better fitness spaces and that there are already amazing people challenging toxic fitness culture and building new communities. This has brought me joy, awareness, reignited purpose, new friendships, and the guilt of not starting my search earlier. I owe almost all the knowledge, language, and courage you can find on these pages to those who have come before me and who have been boldly doing this work even at the cost to their own physical and mental health. It turns out the only barrier keeping me from this reservoir of new role models, relationships, and deep conversations was me.

I am no expert on masculinity, nor do I have the perfect solution for the fitness industry, but I know trauma, I know the power of community, and I am a man who has spent most of his life in gyms. With my knowledge, many privileges, and voice, it is my responsibility to fight for something better. It is precisely because of the protections afforded to me by my identities that I must rise to match the bravery and radical authenticity of those without those protections who are leading the way. The voices of those at the intersections of the harm need to be centered. The people most excluded, oppressed, and judged by the fitness industry (and by the world) are those who know most intimately what needs to change. While it is not the job of the oppressed, specifically, fat, Black, Indigenous, People of Color (BIPOC), Transgender and Gender Non-Conforming, Queer, and Disabled People, to educate everyone else, it is our collective responsibility to listen to the many activists who have been fighting for their existence, humanity, and access.

If we want to see a new culture in fitness, we need to meet the current one just as it is. We need to acknowledge honestly the foundation of white supremacy, patriarchy, and shame-funded capitalism that grounds the fitness-industrial complex in blatantly anti-Black, racist, transphobic, homophobic, sexist, anti-fat, and ableist practices. The sobering truth we must start with is that this culture is toxic to all. It unquestionably harms some more than others, but the fitness industry spares no one. It heals no one, it loves no one, and it relies on shame, competition, domination, and self-hatred to exist.

Our fitness spaces must become more trauma-informed. As a therapist, trust me when I tell you that most of the symptoms people share with me are better understood once a trauma history has been explored. Trauma can be acute, chronic, and complex. Examples of trauma include a near-death experience, an abusive relationship, sexual assault, an oppressive institution, and the loss of a loved one. Trauma has many sources and many definitions, but to me, the hallmark of trauma is any experience resulting in significant emotional impact that one does not currently possess the resources to bear, process, or escape from. Traumatic experiences demand that our bodies and minds adapt to survive. Unfortunately, these adaptions often compel survivors to trade authenticity, trust, relationships, and curiosity for anything that provides an increased sense of safety and control. Trauma can occur at the individual, the community, the system, and the intergenerational level and most often impacts those with intersecting oppressed identities. Fitness spaces, just like relationships, hold incredible potential for both healing and harming people.

The fitness-industrial complex has resulted in widespread personal, complex, and collective trauma. All traumas deeply impact the nervous system and the body. A body too long in survival mode is a body that is slowly poisoning itself. At our core, humans are wired for connection, community, relationships, and resilience. We need other humans to heal, to thrive, and to find meaning.

When I daydream about trauma-informed fitness spaces, I see an untapped goldmine. I envision spaces created for all bodies and centered on the needs of the most vulnerable. Spaces where people feel safe and supported enough to take intentional risks. Where new relationships with others can be explored both authentically and consensually. Where a loving relationship with your body can be prioritized. Where narratives about strength, health, and fitness can be empowering instead of shaming. Where wholeness is valued over perfection and people are valued inherently. Where people can come as they are without being excluded, objectified, sexualized, judged, harassed, exploited, mocked, bullied, or guilt tripped. I have learned that the heart of working with trauma begins in our relationships, within our bodies, and within the narratives we create. These avenues of healing and resilience benefit us all and are possible if we are willing to resist the current status quo.

When I think about that little Alaskan boy shooting bricks into a double-rimmed, chain-netted hoop, there is so much I want him to know. You are loved already and your loving heart is what matters most. For your heart is the bridge. The bridge to community, not competition. To accountability, not apathy. To connection, not isolation. You were made to move and you get to do that in whatever way feels most authentic. There is no right way to be an athlete, other than the right way for you, and you get to be so much more. You are going to hear a lot of ideas about how to be a man. Most of them are bullshit. It is actually more important for you to figure out what it means to be you. And to fight until everyone has that same chance. It is your job to keep fighting no matter how slow the progress, so that those who come after you have fewer barriers, less hate, and more love. You will find far more meaning in advocating for love and justice than you ever will from sports. You will learn that that humility, empathy, and critical thinking do not come easy, yet are so worth it. Instead of trading your integrity for status, or for comfort, you can learn how to let go of your ego and to be accountable for the ways these systems have given you an unfair advantage. In return, you will find growth, connection, and the calm peace of an unconflicted soul. You were put here to hold space, not to take it.

CHAPTER 5

Learning to Love My Body beyond Perception

ADELE JACKSON-GIBSON

One discovers the light in darkness, that is what darkness is for; but everything in our lives depends on how we bear the light. It is necessary, while in darkness, to know that there is a light somewhere, to know that in oneself, waiting to be found, there is a light.

—JAMES BALDWIN, *Nothing Personal* (1964)

1. love as admiration?

In third grade, I discovered what it meant for me to be able to jump far. And I don't mean in feet, meters, or some other physical metric. What I'm talking about is what I—a lankier-than-most Black girl attending a new school full of white kids—found the moment I realized that I had hops: social footing.

It was a sunny spring day in that small gym with blond, creaky flooring. The sun filtered through the large open windows, warming the grassy air while bedazzling the dust. The room echoed with kid laughter and glittered with the promise of something old made new. Our teacher, Mr. Ash—the bodybuilder who could make his pecs dance—was showing us how to do the standing broad jump, now a remnant Olympic track and field event.

He split us into groups as we filed behind the green sidelines. We each took turns practicing the rhythm: squat, launch, plant, then eyeball the distance we had traveled in one lemur leap. The whole time, my body rattled with the anticipation of seeing how far I could go.

When I landed with a bang and a squeak, the room echoed with other sounds I was surprised to hear: "Whoas" and "Wows" from my classmates. This grabbed Mr. Ash's attention, so he came over to watch me leap again. *Bang-squeak!* He smiled and crossed his arms to cradle a prideful chest. This may have been the first time someone called me "athletic."

I knew this to mean being "active or gifted in sports, games, or exercises," as *Merriam-Webster* puts it.[1] Maybe this explained the pure ecstasy I felt trying to run as fast as I could around the neighborhood cul-de-sac, though it's hard to say. After all, you don't have to be "good" at anything to enjoy it, as much as we tend to entangle those two.

What the dictionary certainly doesn't describe, however, is that "athletic" usually means that you'll be liked—or at least be one of the kids who got picked first for kickball at recess. I wasn't cool. But this new description was, for me, a person who struggled to fit into this Catholic school, both a sacred refuge and a cherished key.

"Athletic."

This word would carry me through track and field state championships and Olympic development soccer camps, grant me access to higher education, and provide me many bands of teammates who gave me a sense of belonging (if not BFF-ship).

"Athletic" would be something that suggested my "betterness" over others. It placed me on this hierarchy of bodies, letting me occupy a more visible, celebrated rung in society than those who are considered "less able." And this, admittedly—regrettably—was something I learned to center my identity on. I liked being faster and stronger than others. I liked collecting the faux gold medals, blue ribbons, and plastic trophies my parents would put up someplace where our dog Snowy couldn't chew on them. I liked the praise I received in the local newspaper, and why wouldn't I? I'm a Sagittarius sun and moon. All the accolades and attention, please.

Eventually, it became clear that some people—particularly white people—thought that my body was both an object worthy of marvel and . . . something I couldn't quite put my finger on for some time. Something along the lines of alarm, faintly tracing shame.

I noticed others beginning to project those perceptions on me when I was about fourteen. Puberty came with a period, boobs, and, unexpectedly, visible abs. This seeming clash of masculinity on the brink of "womanhood" was an equation that was hard for some people to compute.

Already feeling unpretty, I didn't necessarily love having extra bulk to call people's attention to how unlike the popular Jennifer Aniston I was (although try spinning around five times, squinting your eyes, and looking at me sideways before you decide). Alas, in the locker room, I'd watch the smoke come out of my classmates' ears as they tried to figure out why my stomach looked the way it did. I must've done sit-ups every day, they said (though I did no more than Coach told us to). I must've skipped out on the donut holes at homeroom, they said (though I most certainly did not). They were so lazy, they'd tell me. If only they weren't so lazy, they'd have muscles. But just toned, you know. Not too muscular because they didn't want to look manly.

Not knowing how to respond to these conversations, I often smiled silently and wondered if I was "too much."

At some point, I started watching pro athletes like Venus and Serena Williams who made me feel way less alien—proud even. It gave me incredible joy to see muscular Black female-identifying athletes taking up white-dominated space. Listening to the way white commentators talked about them, though, made me feel more animal. I'd read about the Williams sisters and how they "destroyed" or "obliterated" their white opponents with their athleticism. I read of tennis fans who called them gorillas, which implied that they were violent, even though gorillas typically are not.

As I continued to follow and participate in sports, I realized that the term *athletic*—especially when it came to describe myself or other Black women athletes—sometimes meant powerful yet unruly; fast but without tact; rough but needing to be refined.

I'm now reminded of historian Amy Bass's essay "Slave Genes Must Die," in which she discussed how sports scientists in the 1930s began comparing white male athletic ability to that of their Black counterparts. Their "studies—which took place in labs at Harvard, Vanderbilt, and Duke—produced some of sport's most venerable racist convictions," Bass wrote in Salon. "Black athletes are more adept at sprinting, more relaxed, make better running backs than quarterbacks, and jump farther, all of which reduced their athleticism to a solely physical condition with no room for intellectual capacity, training nor discipline."[2]

In other words, we were often seen as brutes without brains.

I internalized narratives like this not only from what I heard in the media but from feedback I would get from some of my coaches. I was more "tenacious," more "aggressive," and "less technical" than the other goalkeepers.

Part of me relished being perceived as a bit wild. My opponents got the message that I was no one to mess with. And another part of me was scared of being seen as a monster.

I remember when I was about ten years old playing a soccer game in Akron, New York, a small village of suburbs and farms. I was playing goalkeeper, and toward the end of the match a white girl from the other team was making her way to the net by herself on a breakaway. I was the last line of defense, so I ran at her for the slide tackle. The ball flew away, but she never got up.

Her leg was broken. I was bewildered, never having hurt someone that badly in my life. I was amazed that my body—large, lankier-than-most—could cause such harm.

You may say that a ten-year-old girl being able to smash another's shin bone is . . . terrifying. Or terrific. Awesome. Or awful.

It has me thinking how admiration and fear share a level of intimacy that can keep people at an arm's reach.

At times, I have felt that this pairing has made it challenging to feel close to people and made it easy to feel othered. Like my mom would say, the white boys at school didn't have crushes on my sisters and me because they feared smart, strong Black women. We triggered their insecurities, which says a lot about the fragility of white masculinity. Their fears were utterly based on betterness. So much subconscious bitterness. Some day—my mom was sure—we would meet someone who was ready to embrace all of who we were.

This is all to say that garnering a degree of respect through sports kept this prep school Black girl afloat and even sailing through rough white-cultured waters. At the same time, it kept alive my hunger to discover connections that were much deeper, moored to something beyond physical hierarchy.

It didn't take much to rattle the ladder. To then hang on meant, at times, to dislocate my humanity, flailing to grasp on to a sense of worth.

The underbelly of admiration grumbled with an unsettling question: "Who was I outside of being athletic?"

2. love as dissociation?

There's a level of masochism that I learned to embrace as a soccer goalkeeper through high school and college.

It was that "blood, sweat, and tears" flavored Kool-Aid. The "no pain, no gain" serenades on my pump-up playlists, belting the romance of the future triumphs I would have after so much dedication and sacrifice. (Eminem's "'Till I Collapse" was on repeat frequently.)

I loved feeling sore after a tough lift session and the searing sensation of soap on my turf burns. After preseason training, there was a good chance you could find me in the physical therapy room shouting Billie Withers songs as I endured biting ice baths with a shit-eating grin. Or maybe: taping up sprained thumbs or ankles to keep myself together for the game ahead. God forbid someone else taking my starting spot.

No doubt there was a sort of resiliency I developed playing sports. This skill required a certain degree of dissociation to keep pushing: feeling the pain and yet not being fully present with the consequences. In my mind, you risked for the reward. Dissociation in this sense was a marker of passion to my sport. (Call it love?) I lived to impress people with that resolve.

This mentality took on a whole other level when I turned twenty-four and became serious about CrossFit, a fitness-based sport where competitors sometimes enter what's called that "pain cave" during their intense training sessions. I've been there in its dark, eerily comforting corners. The world is simple there, if not on fire. Some researchers say there's a razor-sharp focus that comes over you under so much physical distress. It provides a space where you can forget about feeling alone, forget about hiding your sexuality, the paper due the following morning. "By flooding the consciousness with gnawing unpleasantness, pain provides a temporary relief from the burdens of self," wrote researchers Rebecca Scott, Julien Cayla, and Bernard Cova.[3] Pain can be intoxicating.

When I moved to New York City to get my master's in journalism, I joined a CrossFit box and started training two times a day. Meanwhile I was working a part-time writing gig, sleeping five hours a night, and fueling myself with protein bars and B12 energy drinks during the workweek, and alcohol and pizza on the weekends.

Balancing this bachelorette-athlete life was thrilling as I was succeeding in work and school. I was also on my way to earning a spot on our gym's regional competition team. It felt like I was constantly sprinting. Or as I would describe it now: perpetually falling, but somehow always catching myself at the right time—until I couldn't.

One Friday, I was finally able to complete 100 butterfly pull-ups during a workout, and afterward was surprised to feel more sore than usual (as if centriplicating an exercise that makes you look like a worm on a hook wasn't peculiar already).

Over the next two days, my biceps became so stiff that I had to massage and yank each arm down just to keep my elbows straight. I laughed at this when I showed my friends, who giggled, "How weird!"

On Sunday, I walked into the gym, smilin', swaggin' like I was Arnold Schwarzenegger at the Olympia. My friends looked at my arms and asked me how I got so swole. The truth: they were swollen, but my balloon head didn't know. Couldn't know. Didn't want to.

But my coach smacked some sense into me when he pulled me aside, looked me dead in the eye, and said: "Adele, your arms look like fucking sausages. You need to go to the hospital, ASAP."

Apparently, he thought I had a condition called rhabdo (aka rhabdo-myolysis), where the body experiences such an excessive amount of muscle breakdown that proteins and electrolytes leak into the blood and can wreak havoc on your organs, particularly your kidneys. The swelling can even cause muscle tissue to die and cause irreversible disability.[4]

"Adele, I'm not joking," my coach said.

I chuckled, thinking my coach was overreacting.

I'd heard of people getting rhabdo in CrossFit, and the symptoms were pretty dramatic like puking, passing out, peeing blood. I had none of that, so I was fine, right? But a blood test at the ER confirmed what my coach had said and that my liver was working overtime to clean up the mess. It was hard for me to swallow the fact that my relationship to pain and suffering was so distorted that I couldn't even tell when my body was on the brink of collapse.

Luckily, my case was mild and I didn't need dialysis (which is what doctors do when the kidneys stop working). Still, over the next three months, the docs sat me in exercise time-out. I couldn't do anything that could potentially make me sore. No long walks, no yoga, and definitely no CrossFit. Not until my lab work was clear.

Day by day, I could feel my bones itching to pick up a barbell, run, or bound up my brownstone's stairs. Feeling like I was useless, a deep sadness blanketed my mind in a suffocating bog. There were days I would lie in bed, letting memories rise to the surface.

I remembered how I had been in this situation before when I'd torn ligaments in my knee and ankle. With each injury came an ego death that was only buried, never laid to rest. Because in the back of my mind I was going to "crush physical therapy" and "return back stronger," ready to hit the ground sprinting all over again.

But this time, the imposed stillness was particularly unsettling for me. It had me come face to face with the fact that for most of my life I had valued myself so much on what my body could do, do, do, that I didn't know how to just be.

So I decided to try out this mantra to lift my spirit: "I am not my body."

I am not my body, but a soul dressed in flesh who happens to like watching anime, telling stories, and singing *NSYNC in the shower; a soul who wants nothing but to share joy with others around her and travel all over the world.

I wrote lists in my head to remind myself that I had meaning outside my body's seeming brokenness. But as much as I tried to separate my body from the aspects that shaped me, each of these things had a corporeality to them that I could not completely slice away. ("What big eyes you have, Adele!" "All the better to watch Naruto with, my dear.")

This mantra—itself an attempt at dissociation—also failed to address the Subconscious Me that didn't seem to live in my mind so much as in my materiality. I'm talking about the me that automatically blinks my eyes to shut out dust or jerks my hand away from the stove that's too hot. The me whose job it is to protect me and keep me alive so I can experience this earth without Conscious Me having to lift too many fingers. It usually finds ways to keep me here, tethered to this earth.

I remember when I snapped my funny bone during a soccer game and how as I laid there on the turf, staring at the cloudy evening sky, Jell-O arm above my head, I couldn't feel a thing. My body had offered me a tender gift. It was as if to say, "You're not ready to feel how fragile you are."

For a moment, I laughed in the lightness of insensitivity, then cried at the realization of what happened. All the while, I was cradled. Held in the palm of numbness to just be.

3. love as self-adoration?

While I healed from rhabdo, I was set on establishing a new relationship with my body and how it factored into the way I related to other people—especially when it came to romance.

Not only was I geared toward using my body as a means to impress and entertain, I had spent years suppressing my sexuality. I knew there were a lot of narratives I internalized about being a Black queer woman that I needed to unlearn before I could be truly present in a relationship. (The story of dykes being ugly being one of them.) I mean, how could I be in touch with my boundaries and desires when I was conditioned to please everyone else before myself? When I was taught that being attracted to women meant I was gross?

I was once told that in order to receive the love you're looking for, you need to first give it to yourself. So after a long spell of being dumped by various not-so-tender Tinder flings and ghosted by okay-daaaaamn-Cupid-why-you-gotta-be-like-thats, I was ready to give this self-love thing a try.

I did all the things many of the self-help gurus prescribed to rewire my brain to the frequency of L.O.V.E.: I looked deep into my eyes in the mirror and repeated affirmations ("I am loving!" "I am loved!"). I drew inspiration from the #bodypositive movement on Instagram (New affirmations! "Black is beautiful!" "Queer is beautiful!" "I am beautiful!"). I tried to keep my outlook as positive as possible, seeing the beauty in everything and everyone. I even listened to feel-good playlists to boost my mood.

Did I end up meeting the love of my life and living happily ever after? Yes, and so far so good. Can I owe all that to imagining Luther Vandross as my Inner Being singing its devoted love to me on my train to work? Lizzo knows.

No doubt fostering more self-love has given me the foundation to further embody and own my authenticity. My queerness. My nerdiness. Never again will I hide my Dragonball Z paraphernalia for seeming uncool.

However, on the days when I was feeling guilty about my anxious skin picking, insecure about the hyperpigmentation dotting my face, or generally angry or sad, my affirmations and mirror work could not hold space for me. On those days, Smash Mouth's "All Star"—a song I tenderly know by heart—sounded like cats fighting in my ears while my other self-love tactics felt like fake-it-until-you-make-its. Sweep-it-under-the-rugs. They kept me in denial about my emotions and thus feeling trapped in a futile battle against myself.

In the realm of social media where we are constantly being fed each other's highlight reels, self-love appears to be this thing where we always have to be happy or at least pursuing happiness. Anything other than "happy" seems unacceptable or something that people would rather not see or hear about. #PositiveVibesOnly. You need to be infatuated with yourself every day no matter how many times heteronormative social and beauty standards push you to the edge. No matter how much that hurts or your body pains you.

No matter how many times that voice in your head tells you to be ashamed for not being this or not being able to do that. Silence it. Sit up tall and say your affirmations louder. Scream them (lovingly, of course): "You are enough! Don't you know you're enough? Know it now. Be it now!"

I admit, this mindset not only made it difficult for me to witness and express my own hurt, disappointment, and frustration, it made it hard for me to witness and accept those emotions in others. Just ask my wife, who in her toughest moments of dealing with her own unique body traumas would get frustrated with me in my rush to "there, there" her. To tell her she was worthy, and beautiful, and everything was going to be okay.

After countless fights and slammed doors, I realized that self-love, at least in the way it was defined in the mainstream, could only get us so far in terms of creating the unconditional support we need individually and collectively. The self-love I was seeing on Instagram reflected adoration, which is cute, but shallow in its depths.

This version of self-love will not carry us through a media culture that tells us that thinner, whiter, and younger is better—that emotions are something for us to abandon. This is partly because this self-love is too focused on changing one's perspective of oneself without acknowledging the various cultural oppressions that influence the self. This is true.

But I also wonder if the problem is also rooted in the way we are defining love. "Love" as "constant adoration" is setting us up for failure. We aren't statues. We are human beings with feelings and sensations that ebb and flow, with lenses of perception that are malleable, with bodies that are constantly changing, reading, adapting, alerting, and protecting, sometimes in ways that we can't appreciate in the moment.

Love to me is not just a feeling but an action. It's dynamic with various components. I like the way the late bell hooks described it in *All about Love*: "To truly love we must learn to mix various ingredients—care, affection, recognition, respect, commitment, and trust, as well as honest and open communication."[5]

What if we took that definition and applied it to self? So rather than thinking of self-love as self-adoration, we thought about it as another opportunity to practice relationship in the way bell hooks envisioned?

Loving our parents, siblings, partner, friends, or dogs is never the same on any given day. Each relationship requires something different at different times with different spirits. And it's not about liking every aspect of them. That does not seem to be required for love. Can't we learn to treat ourselves the same?

Like what if that voice in your head that's tearing you apart is you as a child? You wouldn't necessarily tell that child "F off!" or drown them out with Taylor Swift. You wouldn't necessarily blame the child for having a "bad" attitude either. To me, self-love has become a way for me to listen to the needs beneath the screams: How can I be kind to myself in this moment? Where can I set a boundary with myself or someone else? Etc.

For me, self-love is not just taking selfies when the light is right, but it's often a dizzying dance with my shadows. I trip over my feet, but I'm moving. Finding myself more accepting of my complexities. And on the days when I don't adore myself—on the days I feel shattered—I try to let people who love me show me the mirror. I try to remember that I can't do the healing work alone.

My community is often there for me to witness what I'm not able to see. To show me how all of my pieces, even the most sharp and jagged, fit together.

4. love as integration.

There's a passage in Toni Morrison's *Jazz* that I keep coming back to every so often. It's a scene where the narrator describes a Black couple making love in their New York City apartment.

> It's nice when grown people whisper to each other under the covers. Their ecstasy is more leaf-sigh than bray and the body is the vehicle not the point. They reach, grown people, for something beyond, way beyond and way, way down underneath tissue.[6]

The body is the vehicle and not the point. Not necessarily a machine, but something to get one from A to B. To relay. To connect. There's a refreshing simplicity and yet overwhelming richness in viewing my body this way; to think that maybe the only reason I'm here in the physical is to know and experience all kinds of connection. To feel the peach fuzz on my wife's cheek, grass tickling my feet, ice cream melting on my tongue, and reggae music humming in my bones.

The richness stems from the fact that these connections are happening on all levels, from the micro to the macro to the meta. Sometimes I imagine that each and every one of my trillions of cells have their own consciousness, each having their own jobs to do, communicating via hormones and nerves, living in their own countries and cultures (like the nations of liver or pancreas). That would make me, my body, an amalgamation of communities.

Sometimes I think about all the wisdom, memories, and patterns these cells contain. My mother's and father's DNA and data from generations away. Like the mole that's on my nose. A genetic mutation formed when I was in the womb, I was told. What story does it hold? Or my hazel eyes inherited from some soul that no one in my family can identify. Who were they? What were they like?

I wonder if sometimes in the "random" moments I feel like crying whether the tears are really mine or those that one of my ancestors weren't allowed to shed during dire moments of oppression. That would make me an honored vessel of release. My ancestor's relief. If time isn't linear then I wonder if I can share my laughter with them, too. Share my gratitude. My wildest dreams.

I also think about how I can easily pick up the energy in a room and how that affects me emotionally. How my good friend sometimes feels pain in the same place where others have been hurt. I don't have that superpower, but I subconsciously pick up other people's accents, mannerisms, and catch phrases as if they were my own. You probably do it, too. Scientists say we are all chameleons in that way.[7] I'm not special. Thanks to my wife, I often say "Heeeeey cutie," to every dog I see on the street. It's never really been me to be sweet to every adorable puppy I meet, but I am constantly becoming, integrating my surroundings—the sugar and the salt—whether I'm fully aware of it or not.

What I'm saying is: I no longer think my body is exactly mine. That in deciphering where you or I or we begin it's kind of hard to draw a line.

Love to me now is learning to flow between our perceived separation and the beauty of our diversity with our undeniable one-bodiedness. To somehow appreciate it all.

There may be a larger picture I will never see, but I believe that everything my body has been through—as an athlete, a human—has meaning for not just me but everyone around me. Nothing about me or my experiences is random. Not all of it I like. But through it all I'm learning the depth of this thing called Love, under the covers, beneath the tissue, and beyond perception.

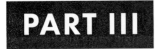

How We Empowered Ourselves to Move Forward and Help Our Communities Polish Their Armor

CHAPTER 6

Landmines

ASHER FREEMAN

It starts in my right hip. But if I miss that signal, I feel it in my knees, bending and straightening like 8,000-year-old hinges with every stair I climb. When I pause for long enough, I feel the inside of my right thigh pulling toward my pelvis, the crease inside of my right leg pulling toward ... And this is where my conscious thought abruptly stops.

◆

I know so many of us have complicated histories in our bodies, so I tread carefully when working with personal training clients. I sense we might be close to a landmine when we are drilling a certain movement pattern and my verbal cues become useless or counterproductive. I say, "Soften your knees," and my client comes into a deep squat. I watch frustration build as bodily awareness tanks.

Sometimes the danger zones are less obvious. After a few weeks of working with a newer client on core engagement, I reintroduced the practice of a pelvic tilt on the ground. I watched her lie on her back, knees bent with her feet on the floor as she tucked her tailbone under. I saw the space between her low back and the floor disappear, a sign that she successfully, intentionally engaged her abdominal muscles. But before I could respond with affirmation, I saw tears streaming down her face. Sometimes this same scene with a different person ends in nausea. For many of my clients, abdominal muscle engagement can unearth carefully tucked-away memories as the stomach recalls years of sucking in that coincided with shame and self-harm.

For clients with similar identities to my own, it can be easier for me to guess when we are venturing into a more emotionally charged part of the body. At this point in my career, I am surprised when trans masculine people can easily feel their chest muscles working. When I ask where they feel a bench press, I expect to hear about many places in their arms and shoulders, but the chest is usually a big blank space. While many of us who have had top surgery have some change in sensation post operatively, surgery alone cannot explain our inability to connect with the muscles in our chest. I have witnessed this same phenomenon in people who have not had surgery and people who had surgery over a decade ago. The only commonality I can discern is some history of dysphoria that creates dissonance between our neuromuscular connections and our conscious awareness.

◆

The tension that comes from a tightly wound ball of avoidance has traveled down from my knees to my ankles and my big toe on the left side. Until I can focus on this knot long enough to understand how and where it is tied, I do not know if this new pain in my wrist is also its doing.

Avoidance multiplies. If I do not interrogate the source of this tension, I worry I cannot understand what harm it is causing. But I do not turn over any stone because I am scared by what I might find underneath.

I've heard more than once that I should sit with discomfort, but how? When the discomfort makes me suddenly disappear from my body, how do I stay?

◆

I have been working with one client on a hinge movement pattern for months. We started on the floor with glute bridges. Lying on his back, he felt the ground give him the support and feedback he needed to keep a long spine. We transitioned to a standing exercise using dumbbells. A few weeks ago, I introduced a barbell deadlift for the first time, and I watched him struggle to keep his spine from curving forward while preparing to pick the bar up from the floor. I tried to help him find a safer position using different prompts. "Lengthen your spine." "Bring your shoulders back." "Try opening your chest."

Eventually he said, "I don't think I can physically do it." Although I have seen him do the same exact movement with different equipment, I did not push the issue.

Even people who have never stepped foot inside of a gym are familiar with phrases like "No pain, no gain," which reflect the dominant fitness industry ideology that ignoring our bodies' limits will somehow make us stronger. In order to gain strength, we do need to challenge ourselves to do more than what is familiar and easy, but we also need to work within the limits of what feels safe. Trauma therapists talk about this in-between space for our nervous system as being our "window of tolerance." I have made the mistake of drilling an exercise for too long in the past. When I push someone past their window of tolerance, their form usually deteriorates with each repetition. Any feedback or suggestions I share once someone has checked out of their body further reinforce a sense of overwhelm and failure.

So when my client said, "I don't think I can physically do it," I listened. We moved to seated overhead presses. I knew this was an exercise he could do well with little thought, an exercise that could help bring him back into his body.

When we met the following week, he was ready to return to the barbell deadlift, and he found the length in his spine without any guidance. After he completed a set of ten, I asked him how they felt.

"Good?" he responded hesitantly, looking for validation that what he felt in his body matched what I witnessed as I watched him move.

"They were beautiful."

He is on his way to a movement practice that does not rely on external feedback. Until then, I can stay by his side, reminding him that his body is smart. Sometimes we need a break from focusing on certain physical sensations. Often, when we listen and allow ourselves to pause, we gain a sense of self-trust and safety that allows us to venture a little further next time.

I consciously relax my glutes, but I feel them squeeze whenever I stretch the front of my hips. I try to breathe in and release with my exhale. Immediately, I notice that familiar knot reaching straight from between my legs to my stomach, making me want to vomit or shut down. I choose to shut down.

During my early twenties, I would spend at least an hour every day lying on the floor. I would be so debilitated and overwhelmed by sharp pains in my stomach that all I could do was stare at the ceiling, waiting for them to dissipate. It would be years until I recognized that this was a problem. Only then did I make the connection between my stomachaches and the bottomless cups of coffee that I drank to keep up with my unmanageable schedule. I found shelter in a demanding workload that shielded my attention from the ever present discomfort that had grown deep roots inside of me.

My coping mechanisms had no contingency plan, however, when I unexpectedly experienced a brutal job loss in my midtwenties. Suddenly, I no longer had a job title or overtime hours to hide behind, and the unease that had taken root throughout my nervous system quickly grew from a distant buzzing to an all-consuming alarm.

In a floundering attempt to turn down the volume on my discomfort, I decided to try out weight lifting for the first time. Being newly unemployed, I bounced from one free gym trial to the next, attempting to soak in as much information from the complimentary one-on-one personal training sessions as I could about weight lifting equipment and exercises. I tried to incorporate all of it into daily workouts. I was getting some ideas about what the exercises were supposed to look like, but it was much more challenging to get a sense of what they should feel like.

I have always been physically active—I grew up playing soccer, and I have been a bike commuter since I was nineteen. However, all the exercises that I loved in my youth and early twenties centered on gross motor skills and required little attention to the technicalities of movement. I could bike, run, and kick without ever paying attention to how or what I was moving. My mind was most at ease whenever I was pushing my body to its limits, or more accurately, ignoring its limits. When my heart was pounding hard enough, it could almost overpower the constant drone of discomfort.

Resistance training requires an awareness of how every part of the body moves through space. It necessitates a presence of mind to stabilize some muscle groups while moving others. For one hour every day, I went to the gym, and I explored what it meant to be in my body. While it would be some time before I began hormones and had top surgery, I mark the beginning of my physical transition with the start of my resistance training.

I remember sitting on a hip adductor machine soon after I began strength training, squeezing my thighs together against the resistance of the pads, when I felt the muscles of my pelvic floor engage for the first time. It felt like a sharpened pencil was pushing itself inside of me. The pulling at my center turned to nausea, shooting up to my stomach and then my throat. My memory fails when I try to retrieve the following moments of this scene. The next recollection I have is standing outside the gym in silence, the sounds of nearby cars and people unable to penetrate the glass walls that had sprung up around me.

I had uncovered a massive landmine, and I had zero tools to address it. I knew I never wanted to feel that way again. At the same time, strength training was one of the few anchors steadying my ego during a demoralizing job search. I needed attainable, straightforward goals like lifting heavier weights to give me a sense of control and accomplishment. On a deeper level, I was beginning to discover what it might feel like to have a more integrated relationship with my body. The warmth of my back muscles contracting as I pulled a dumbbell toward my chest allowed me to be firmly in the present, providing a brief respite from my lifelong desperation to escape. I was not ready to process my experience on the hip adductor machine, so I chose to continue weight lifting as if it never happened.

Looking back, there was another layer that drew me to the gym initially. I wanted the same thing that many of my trans masculine clients tell me they are seeking: wider shoulders and narrower hips. Due to my extreme stubbornness, and perhaps acting on some internalized transphobia, I was intent on "doing the work myself" without the help of medical interventions. I recorded videos to track physical changes and gave myself one year to make the changes myself before deciding whether to go on testosterone.

Inevitably, I learned that genetics and hormones determine much more about body composition and fat distribution than I ever could with exercise. But while strength training did not significantly change how my body looked, it completely overhauled my relationship to my body. Watching my videos now, I see my younger self growing confidence and a hard-earned sense of bodily autonomy. By the time I sought out a testosterone prescription, I did not do it because I failed at building enough muscle mass. I started testosterone because I had begun to inhabit my body more fully, and I understood that hormones were the right next step for me.

◆

When I'm still, meaning when my body is still and my brain is elsewhere, my pain might go down to a one or a two. The second I tune in to the spark in my knee, my nervous system clicks on and I feel electricity everywhere. When I stand, I feel the tension screaming from the front of my ankles to the swelling that erupts from the right side of my back, and every muscle that originates at my right hip lights up.

◆

I spent the first decade of my adulthood working with youth and as a community organizer in jobs that enabled me to focus my attention and compassion outward. During those years, I asked an endless stream of open-ended questions to others without ever pausing to consider or share my own responses. As I approached my thirtieth birthday, I noticed that the anxious energy that coursed through my veins was beginning to wane. By that point, I had changed my name and pronouns and begun my medical transition. As the deep discomfort in my bones began to settle, I found myself wanting to decrease the distance between my inner life and the world around me.

I was ready to find a job that fit well with my life and not the other way around. I made a list of qualities I wanted in a job: I wanted to do more good than harm; I wanted to build deep one-on-one supportive relationships with people; and I wanted to move my body. In order to reach those goals, I became a full-time student in an exercise science program while continuing to work full-time as a community organizer. Ironically, as I began working toward a future career devoted to embodiment and connectedness, I once again turned off any cues from my body of discomfort or pain.

There have been few periods in my life in which I exercised less than while I was studying to become a personal trainer. My body floated from campus to my office to the apartment complexes where I was doing tenant organizing to the state capital where we were fighting for legal reform. That familiar pulse of adrenaline in my veins, paired with caffeine, fueled me far more than food or water that year. During spring break, I had top surgery and completely ignored my surgeon's guidance to take a few weeks off from work and school. I remember dragging my body around the city the following week, tubes still hanging from my fresh incisions as blood pooled in the drains that were pinned to the inside of my shirt. Finally, I collapsed on the couch and realized that I was physically unable to get up.

A few months after I was cleared by my surgeon to exercise, and as my college program was winding down, I devised a plan. I would finish the program, leave my job, and depart the following week to move cross-country from Portland, Oregon, to Philadelphia. By bicycle.

In the full-throttle mode of my life, it made perfect sense. I was moving to live with my partner. I had dreamt of biking across the country for years, and this was the first time I would not have a job or a job search preventing me from taking the time needed to make the trip. My friend and I were the last cyclists of the season to ride east on the Trans America route.

We started our ride on August 15, knowing that we needed to move quickly and get lucky to miss the snow in the Rockies and arrive in time for an important family commitment. We rode eight hours a day for sixty-five days. We biked until we were too tired to do anything other than set up camp, cook food, and pass out. We took a total of seven days off. And we arrived at the Chesapeake Bay seventy-three days and 4,300 miles later.

I left for the bike tour about a month after I became a certified personal trainer, yet I convinced myself it was okay for me to skimp on rest days and essentially skip stretching during a two-and-a-half-month-long bike ride. I had seamlessly transitioned from my mentally strenuous work-and-school marathon to the extreme physical exertion I first learned as a kid. I felt high biking over the Continental Divide, two miles above sea level, and sprinting to race my friend to each sign marking our entry into a new state or county. I cannot remember being so free from anxiety as I was during those months on my bicycle. However, I was about to learn once again that the ecstasy that I experienced when ignoring my body's physical limits came with a price.

During the first week of our tour, while still in Oregon, I developed a minor knee injury, likely due to a total lack of training prior to leaving. I iced my knee a few times and then turned to ibuprofen as my sole recovery tool while I pedaled along. "I'll deal with it when I get to Philadelphia," I told myself.

It may have been possible to fully recover from my injury after my bike tour. I certainly knew from my exercise science program that the sooner I treated my injury, the better my recovery would be. Instead of treatment, however, I became a runner. The emotional comedown from my tour coupled with being underemployed and anonymous in a new city left me feeling deeply uncomfortable. For a quick fix, I once again turned the intensity up louder than my discomfort. I began running five miles a day. I had not run for exercise since middle school, but it was the only form of movement that was capable of quieting my mind and staving off the depression that I could feel lurking just out of sight.

After a few weeks of running, I could no longer ignore the pain in my knee. I lost the ability to go up stairs, and walking became incredibly painful.

I wrap my fingers tightly around the cold metal bar above me. I feel anticipatory warmth spread across my chest where I once felt nothing. The excitement travels through the front of my shoulders and down my arms. Energy from the weight of this bar pulls my consciousness into my physical form.

Eventually, my injury forced me to slow down. I began months of physical therapy while simultaneously starting to work with clients for the first time as a personal trainer. I tried to push through pain in order to demonstrate exercises at work. However, some days I had no choice but to surrender to my body's demands. I had to admit to my clients that I was not able to bear weight on a bent leg as I verbally cued them through exercises.

It took time, in a new city as a new trainer, to find enough work, and my knee injury meant I could not return to my familiar coping mechanism of extreme physical exertion. I fell into a depression deeper than any I had experienced since high school. I spent more time alone than I ever had. The familiar buzzing sensation became slower and heavier than before, settling into my chest and throat.

My work was the one thing that forced me out of my home. I took the bus for an hour each way to a box gym where I had a three-hour shift, making $7.25 an hour. The majority of the other trainers were cisgender men twice my size. All of them misgendered me, and some gave me fist bumps and used an excessive amount of "man" and "bro" in a clumsy attempt to hide their discomfort. After my shifts ended, I was reluctant to return to the isolation of my apartment but did not have money or reason to travel elsewhere. I made myself a fortress of free weights and resistance bands, tuned out the overpowering masculinity around me, and turned my attention to my own workout. I had to be thoughtful about how I moved my body and pay attention to its signals so as not to aggravate my knee injury. Eventually, I found my way back into a resistance training practice that grounded me.

It took about a year of rehab until my knee was ready to squat with weight. In that time, I was forced to change how I relate to my body once again. In physical therapy, I revisited exercises I had long ago written off as too easy. Slowing them down to focus on my form was humbling. Performing simple bodyweight exercises meant I could no longer measure my success externally with the amount of weight on my bar. I had to tune back in to how my body was moving through space rather than what it was moving.

When I lost the ability to drown out my discomfort, I had to sit in it. I certainly did not heal every pain in that year, but I learned that it was possible to heal. I was finally ready to do this work. I had dipped my toes in when I began weight lifting, but I did not have the internal resources then to stay with my discomfort.

Even now, I have blank spaces, physical locations in my body where I cannot let my attention rest. I have stones that I am not ready to turn over. However, because of how far I have come and because of the growth I get to witness in my clients, I know that recovery in our relationships to our bodies is possible. We need time and an abundance of patience to move at the pace of our own healing.

The tightness in my right hip is glowing red and warm. I breathe into it and try to relax with a long exhale. The feeling does not dissipate, but it also does not intensify. Now I notice my left forearm. It is completely still, getting heavier and tingly as my attention lingers. It is light blue and cool. I breathe in and, with my exhale, I invite the hazy light blue border to grow a few centimeters. I see the blue and the red, the parts that are healed and the parts I have yet to untangle.

CHAPTER 7

Reframing Pilates to Meet Our Bodies

SONJA R. PRICE HERBERT

I never really thought about it until now, but I was born in 1968, three years after the Jim Crow laws were abolished. These were state and local laws enforcing racial segregation that existed from 1877 to 1965. That means four generations of my ancestors all lived underneath these laws. I, along with my brothers born in 1965 and 1971, barely escaped by a few years, though we felt the aftershock of integration in our hometown of Paris, Texas.

On my birth certificate, my parents and I were classified as "Negro." I remember my mother telling me that the doctors were not sure who my father was because I was so fair skinned. My older brother and mother were much darker than me. Once my father, also fair skinned, arrived to see me, the question was answered. My light skin didn't get me much of anything in school because white people still called me the N-word. I noticed the lack of Black teachers and representation very early in my life but was not sure what I could do about it. Black people were conditioned to believe that there was nothing you could do. This was the world as we see it, and to complain would mean you were not satisfied with what you have already.

It would be many years later that my Negro skin would show up in a different way within the fitness industry. I never expected it actually. My understanding of racism and white supremacy was still developing, and as I look back, there were many things I missed because my eyes were not open nor was I knowledgeable about microaggressions. Fitness was supposed to be a safe space for everyone. It was a space where I could experience my truest self and how best to care for myself individually. It was where I would develop confidence. Nothing would prepare me for the stark reality that I would face upon the beginning of Pilates certification.

Joseph Pilates started "the art of control or contrology" in Germany. As a young boy he struggled with asthma and rickets yet was still quite the athlete. He began rehabilitating immobile World War II soldiers by attaching springs to the bed. This made it easier for those soldiers to go through rehabilitation without actually having to leave their beds. It worked, and Mr. Pilates found himself continuing to advance upon his method. He eventually moved to the United States, where he started the first studio in New York City along with his wife Clara Pilates. He would work with everyone from business people to housewives to singers, dancers, and other artists. Kathleen Stanford Grant, a Black dancer, would be his first and only Black client. Ms. Grant would continue his work by managing her own studio at the now defunct Henri Bendels. Through Ms. Grant, many Black celebrities, dancers, and everyday people would be introduced to the method of contrology but with a Black face. She made it accessible to many Black dancers who did not have the funds to pay for sessions. Some of those dancers were her very first assistants, Wendy Amos, Dr. Jacqueline Sawyer, and Sarita Allen, who would learn under her tutelage without the restraint of financial hardship. Ms. Grant would become mother, mentor, and friend to them and others until her death May 27, 2010.[1]

Living as an adult in New York City, I was performing in off-Broadway musicals and taking on a few singing gigs here and there. My daughter was dancing at Harlem School of the Arts. There, I would find out about a thing called Pilates. A dance teacher friend had told me about the class. I had never heard of it but decided to try it since Cynthia Shipley (my daughter's dance teacher) was teaching the class. After one class, I found myself going twice a week. I wanted to learn more and eventually spoke to Ms. Shipley about becoming a teacher. In 2007 I completed my mat certification at a certification studio in downtown New York. During my certification, I was the only Black apprentice. Once I completed my comprehensive certification in 2008 and started teaching regularly, I began to notice that there were not very many Black Pilates teachers. One of my teacher trainers was a Black woman and so was Ms. Shipley, but beyond them, I rarely saw myself.

I was the only Black Pilates apprentice in my certification. In the world of Pilates, it was expected that you would eventually have a "Pilates body," which consisted of long, lean muscles with no bulk. This was how we were to describe and sell Pilates to customers. I worked at the front desk as part of the work study program. It was rare I ever saw any client who looked like me. The majority of this studio's clientele were white. They had what appeared to be the type of body Pilates could give, or at least they were working toward that. In fact, I cannot remember if I ever saw someone with a larger body attend any classes. As I reflect back, I realize that the marketing of their particular Pilates style was directed at white, thin people who could do the exercises as taught.

After every class, clients would talk about much their body had changed but only from an aesthetic point of view. Pilates had helped them lose weight, tone their arms, and get flat abs. Again, I was still maturing and did not realize that right before my eyes I was being enveloped into the fitness-industrial complex. Pilates had become this elite exercise model specifically for those who wanted a particular body. Joseph Pilates, creator of the method, describes Pilates in his book *Pilates' Return to Life through Contrology* as "the complete coordination of body, mind and spirit."[2] He goes on to also say that "Pilates (originally called Contrology) develops the body uniformly, corrects postures, resources physical vitality, and invigorates the mind, and elevates the spirit." Nothing in that description says long, lean muscles or weight loss. Perhaps that person did not begin Pilates to lose weight; however, it was certainly something regularly discussed in client circles as well as among instructors.

I did not feel entirely immersed in the fitness industry, as Pilates had its own subculture, until I started working for Equinox. As a niche luxury gym, they catered to the elite, wealthy, and white. It was apparent in their marketing. Thin bodies and luxury life mean great health. I remember their first Pilates marketing commercial. There were about four white instructors on reformers in a circle. It was apparent that neither I nor anyone who did not fit that aesthetic was welcome. In my five years of employment, I learned that as much as management celebrated our sales victories, they were not concerned about my individual health. It was all about serving their customers. Some would say it is a niche; I would say it is purposeful exclusion for the sake of monetary exchange. The color of my skin was not enough to capitalize on.

Pilates at Equinox was equally exclusionary as it was in a studio, but just on a wider spectrum. Of all my regular clients, only two of them were Black. By the time they had started working with me, I had already dispelled the long, lean body myth, and neither of those clients even mentioned wanting that result. I found it interesting that my white clients expected this result while the Black clients did not. Perhaps it was because Pilates was always touted as an exercise method for white people, so we were not privy to its reputation as a specific body type.

I would eventually audition to teach mat Pilates for Equinox's group fitness program. I received a standing ovation after my audition and was told that my class was by far the most difficult. Within a week, I received an email from the group fitness manager saying that they loved me but felt I was too aggressive in my teaching style although I was the best out of everyone. He said they wanted me to audition again and "tone it down." I told my new Pilates manager and another coworker (she got hired; she was also white) who auditioned with me what I was told. They were appalled. I decided at that point I would not do anything other than teach private Pilates sessions for Equinox.

I met Dyane Harvey-Salaam, dancer, choreographer, and co-founder of Forces of Nature Dance Theater, in 2010. This meeting would be the catalyst to my work as an activist for Black equity and justice in the Pilates industry. Dyane had worked with Kathy Grant and was in the process of starting a group called Pilates Instructors of Color (PIC). I had expressed to her my idea of starting a group for Black Pilates instructors but felt I was not the one to lead the group at that time. That is when she told me about the PIC group and invited me to one of the meetings. I first learned about Kathy Grant from Dyane and later a much deeper history from Sarita Allen, a former Alvin Ailey dancer and mentee of Kathy's. Kathy had died a few months before I met Dyane, who had also invited me to attend the memorial service where I would meet more Black instructors she had impacted. I was not able to attend but did get a chance to attend the PIC meetings. Due to schedule conflicts, we disbanded.

In 2017 the Black community was experiencing a lot of police brutality resulting in protests in cities across the United States. At that same time, I felt the need to be among my community in Pilates, but it was rare that I met anyone. During what was one of the darkest times of my life, I decided to create what I could not find. I knew we had to be somewhere but needed to be found. Racism seemed so clear in the Pilates method, and surely I was not the only one feeling excluded because of my Blackness.

On May 27, 2017, I founded Black Girl Pilates, a collective of Black-identifying women who taught Pilates. Three years later, I would find out that this was ten years to the day that Kathy Grant passed away. Perhaps this was some sort of way Kathy was speaking to me, but it definitely made me feel like she was my guardian angel. Within one day, I had added fifty women to my Facebook support group. Word spread about this "affinity" group, but not everyone was excited about it. I was called "racist and divisive," and an instructor said I needed to "get my head checked." White instructors attempted to join the support group and accused me of discrimination due to the color to their skin. Interesting that they would play the reverse racism game, as Black instructors had been experiencing this all of their lives in every facet of life. An antiracism educator, Catrice Jackson, had been working with *Girls Gone Strong (GGS)*, a platform that I followed for fitness information. She had said they were looking for some Black writers and asked if I was interested. My first article, "Let's Talk about Black Female Representation in Fitness," for *GGS* was published the weekend before the Ferguson protest. It could not have been published at a better time. After that I continued to write for *GGS* as well as *Self* magazine and a few other platforms about representation, racism, and white supremacy.

After my first few experiences of racism from white Pilates instructors, I realized this was a much bigger issue that I had not paid very much attention to. I had also gaslit myself, saying that much of what happened was not based on race. Yet there was a certain part of me who knew that it was racially based. I had heard many stories from the folks in my group of racism, discrimination, microaggressions, and elitism. I knew then that I needed to do much more than use the Black Girl Pilates platform for representation. Black people cannot be represented until white folks acknowledge that they refused to see us. Our voices were never at the table, and we were not asked to sit at those seats unless that meant the white agenda would continue. We needed more than just our faces. I was determined to speak out against the injustices within the Pilates method. Of course, I was met with gaslighting and blatant racism. It did not stop the group from growing. By August, I had 150 members in the group. In October 2017 we had our first "meet up" in New York City. It was amazing meeting the folks you only knew from Instagram or Facebook. Many of us had shared racist incidences that we thought were just our own personal experiences, only to find it was happening industry-wide. As we became more visible, membership continued increasing. Still, representation in the industry at large didn't budge.

The attention on Black Lives Matter, police brutality, and racial inequality in June 2020 sparked an uprising in the Black Pilates community against the powers that be that continued to gatekeep and promote anti-Blackness, racism, and elitism. My call to action became more than holding Pilates organizations accountable for their anti-Black behavior. I created my first antiracism webinar for the Pilates community called "Introduction to Anti-racism for Pilates Studios and Instructors." The response was overwhelming and much greater than I expected.

I also knew that this would only be a trend and eventually these responses would weaken as the hashtags grew fewer. I would find other ways to educate, like the Decolonizing Pilates Mentorship Program, a three-month-long intensive for white Pilates instructors. Not only would they examine and re-examine their racist conditioning but be taught by some of the best Black Pilates instructors in the industry. Many had **NEVER** been taught by a Black instructor in their career. The founding group completed a book discussion on *Do Better: Spiritual Activism for Fighting and Healing from White Supremacy* by my longtime friend Rachel Ricketts. At the end of the course, they raised $5,000 for her to come and speak to the group. Since that time, I have mentored two instructors and hosted four other mentorship programs, started a membership forum for white instructors to continue to grow in their antiracism journey, and wrote my first book, called *The Antiracism Affirmation Guide*.

I am presently pursuing my master of social work degree and plan to open a Pilates studio that will include a clinical practice specifically for Black women and girls. This would give me the chance to do everything I love for a community that I love.

I have had **MANY** times when I wanted to give up and just felt completely burned out. I wondered if my work was impactful or even worth the sacrifices I have made. I realized that it is not up to me to change white people's minds about Black people; it is up to them to hear us and make the change because Black people deserve it.

CHAPTER 8

Fitness of the Soul

SUNAINA RANGNEKAR

Beloved reader, I hope this text may lead you in more sincere devotion, dedication, and direction toward Vaikunta—the spiritual heaven that holds the liberation of all bodies.

This is not just about the fitness-industrial complex but about much more. We must dissect the binaries that create these standards constantly validated and reinforced by society, causing confusion, conflict, and mental affliction. We deserve more. These systems that analyze and critique our bodies are political and ingrained into us from a very young age. So it is not a surprise we find ourselves questioning our understanding of why this confusion, conflict, and affliction exist—gaslighting our oppression! They label us lazy, unhealthy, or unfit to be parents, which is precisely calculated to degrade our self-esteem. The reality is: every single body, including yours, deserves love, freedom, acceptance, and above all, autonomy.

Yoga comes from the root word *Yuj*, meaning "unity" or "oneness." To be one, we must be present. If we can simply be present, perhaps we won't need anything else. As the first line of Patanjali's Yoga sutras state:

अथ योगानुशासनम्

"Atha Yoga Anuśāsanam"

"Now the Teachings of Yoga Begin"

My orientation to this work is from a queer, non-binary yoga student and guide's lens. However, this was not always the lens I saw Yoga through. After accepting myself and incorporating all these nontraditional aspects of my identity, I began seeing a different pattern than society had fed me. Looking into my past experiences with Yoga, I understood that it plays a significant role in how I now show up in Yoga spaces. Through this process of unraveling, I received clues as to how I can alchemize these experiences to create a better future for myself and other yoga practitioners.

What does the "perfect" Yoga body look like? How does it practice Yoga? Is it thin, flexible, strong yet limber? Can it stand, walk, climb stairs, and do all the "normal" things you expect from practitioners? Does it get injured or sick? Does a Yoga practitioner only focus on asana—the physical movement of Yoga?

Every Body Is a Yoga Body!

I continually remind myself that Yoga, like fitness, shows itself in many forms. The definition of fitness cannot be simplified as active, vigor, or able-bodied. The body and mind are only part of what we are. The body and mind are almost always accounted for in the fitness world. But what can be said about the fitness of the Soul? The fitness of the Soul is unchanging. From the Bhagavad Gita, I learned that a Soul cannot be touched by any element, nor can it ever be destroyed. It's beyond the material; it is the goal of Yoga that is rarely discussed within western Yoga spaces. Yoga has been diluted to the point of being unrecognizable. I can't count how many times I have heard "It is the light within me that sees and honors the light within you." But, somehow, they can't see my color, race, sexuality, or gender. While change is constant, we must do our duty to not be a passerby when this kind of harm happens. We must minimize harm, even if that means disrupting a system that infringes on the health and happiness of all.

Yoga is meant to bring us into the present moment. I struggled with this as I stepped into white-owned Yoga studios populated by thin, white, able-bodied women in tight yoga clothes. Yet despite what these spaces tell me, I know that Yoga is not limited to "full extension of the pose" or being able to do a handstand. Yoga is more than asana. Although they may face some of the same life obstacles that I do, their experience is not that of a brown, hairy, non-binary person who has no plans on being digestible to the western public. Still, the same Self that resides in me is also in them and everyone. However, there are many obstacles to realizing and understanding the true nature of this eternal Self.

My trans body is a vehicle
Transporting my Soul from place to place
In this realm and in the astral.
I feel a block,
Is this because of my skin, my race?
Where does this live in my body?
Inhale to that space
Exhale to ground your place
BAM!
Obstacle: Vyadhi—material body.
Deterioration. Pain. Grief.
In comes comments on my body
Suddenly I can't breathe.
I watch myself dying slowly.
Depressed. Ruled by emotions.
Playing the scene again and again.
I am not my feelings.
I am not my feelings!
BAM!
Obstacle: Styana—mental stagnation or agitation.
So what?! Who cares?!
It happened once,
and it will happen again.

But, it won't stop me from living my life.

Here comes fight, flight, freeze

and worse of all these:

Fawn.

I can do it later.

Deadlines are my biggest enemy.

My mind is my frenemy.

Do I trust my mind, or is it tricking me?

BAM!

Obstacle: Samsaya—doubting what IS.

This can't be it.

So naive to the purpose of it all.

Why must I suffer? Why me?

Imagining all the ways I could be,

the ways I should be.

BAM!

Obstacle: Pramada—carelessness.

How can I be responsible for my thoughts?

Those are definitely beyond me!

Bypassing responsibility for me.

To be proud of who I am—

I connect with the true nature of my being,

with stillness, with silence.

Reminding me: I am doing enough.

I am ENOUGH.

BAM!

Obstacle: Alasya—laziness.

Not rest. More like avoiding my work.

Overwhelmed with emails, texts,

DMs, and various calendar events.

I have enough to do.

Still, I cannot sleep.

BAM!

Obstacle: Avirati—the flood of desire/craving.

I'm overstimulated, and my brain wants more.

More affirmation! More validation!

Obsessing over my Body.

Pushing my Body.

BAM!

Obstacle: Bhrantidarsana—extreme perspectives.

"You can't practice AHIMSA without being vegan, of course." "You can't prac-
tice Yoga without asana."

"There is only one right way, and that's my way!"

Unable to see

the infinite ways water finds its way

back to sea.

Stuck in one way.

BAM!

Obstacle: Alabhdabhumikatva—inability to move to the next step.

What I don't resolve today

waits for me tomorrow.

If I ignore the lesson at hand

the same lesson follows.

Asserting itself in new ways

'til I embody the wisdom and

use it to shape my tomorrows.

BAM!

Obstacle: Anavasthitattva—tendency to backtrack.

I learned the lesson, and still, I relapse

Back to the safety of habits.

Not 'cause I'm less than.

But because

sometimes lessons take lifetimes.

Understand these obstacles, and know that you **CAN** and **WILL** overcome each one with discipline and discernment. Asana improves the conditions of your mind and body to create more peace, understanding, and compassion for yourself and others. To calm the mind and body. Giving us space to know the true Self and the union of the eternal being you are. It may not happen in this life or in this moment. With humility, we can witness that we are all reflections of one another. This is Yoga stripped of Western distortion.

I experienced my first "Yoga class" in seventh grade with my white friend and her mother in Boulder, Colorado. I remember a Ganesha painted on the wall outside the dressing room and the teacher pushing the class to chant in Sanskrit without explaining the mantra. All this while pouring sweat in a 100-degree room for over an hour and a half. Hosting classes on Yoga for six-packs, toning bodies, or losing weight. These kinds of Yoga spaces caused more separation in me than unity. I left feeling less than, comparing my stiff seventh-grade body to that of some able-bodied contortionist who was most likely doing Yoga-asana longer than I had been alive.

When we approach Yoga without acknowledging its roots, we deny each other authenticity and safety. I was exposed to microaggressions, exploitation, and fetishization in Yoga spaces like this. I didn't feel that Yoga spaces could provide safety for me to show up with all my identities. Too often, I witnessed folks using Yoga to actively cause harm, distorting its meaning to fit their own agenda. This able-bodied version of Yoga in the west is maintained at an institutional level through organizations like Yoga Alliance. So how can a white-owned European company decide who receives Yoga teacher certifications? Who decided that they were the authority in Yoga?

For years, I lifted up and centered teachers like this and forfeited my culture and heritage. At the time, I was unaware that I had been practicing Yoga for many years. It is ingrained in every detail of my culture. And while that moment initiated my search for acceptance, I lost myself again. I was looking for validation and grasping for perfectionism in a practice I had unknowingly embodied my entire life.

Almost ten years later, I found my community of South Asian, Black, and queer/trans teachers. I learned about the Yamas and Niyamas—the core ethics that shape Yoga. With this knowledge and community, I could reshape my practice and take accountability for how I had perpetuated harm in Yoga. It's not easy to reflect on how each of us has created harm. It will bring up unpleasant feelings, memories, and fears. But in the end, these things help us grow and shed light on the shadow self. Once I could address how I created harm, I could move forward in a way that would help others like me alchemize their experiences, polish their armor, and become beacons of safety and union.

My practice has heavily shaped my understanding of art, creativity, poetry, and much more. Poetry allowed me to dive deeper into knowing the eternal nature of myself through the obstacles I face. I need to know what I am to know what I am not. Neti Neti, "Not this and not this either."

FROM "MINORITY" TO GLOBAL MAJORITY: an evolution of vernacular

Black, Indigenous, & People of Color
Many call me: BIPOC.
FACT:
We folks of color are the majority of the world!
We are never minor . . . Only MAJOR!
Us, the minority?
Just another white lie.
We are growing.
We are GROWING.
And soon, we will all be different shades of honey.
A magnificent vibrant rainbow of every shade of brown.
I AM THE GLOBAL MAJORITY. Don't call me BIPOC.

I often need to remind myself that we are **THE GLOBAL MAJORITY**. There's nothing minor about us. Ancient practices exist throughout the many cultures of the global majority to connect us to The **ALL** through the physical, mental, and emotional bodies. This is Yoga, and it is also fitness. The more you practice, the easier that connection comes.

THE LAST THING TO GO

The hair on my legs was long.
Armpits dyed purple, wispy, glowing in the sun.
A happy-trail blazed
resting freely on my lower stomach
beneath my crop top.

After 22 years,
My eyebrows grew wild.
I stopped threading them.
I released my crutch
and
let go of the story.
The child of an eyebrow threader
modeling an exquisite unibrow.
Reclaiming their energy
that had been exponentially halved.

A fantastically hairy,
Non-binary goddexx flowered!
Walking this earth in all of their glory
With divine grace
Blessed by their Transcenstors to show up
Exactly
As
They
Are!

CHAPTER 9

On Leaving the Fitness-Industrial Complex

BECK M. BEVERAGE

When I talk to Justice Williams, founder of Fitness 4 All Bodies, he encourages me to "dig up the roots" of my wants, needs, thoughts, and desires. Can we continue doing "fitness," being "fitness professionals," and not have our feet rooted in cultural agreements that are inherently oppressive? Personally, I don't think so.

Most of my seven years as a personal trainer, and then studio owner, were spent trying to figure out how to do fitness in a way that truly aligned with my values. Through my own independent practice and serving as witness to other people's processes, I became increasingly disillusioned. I felt frustrated by the constraints created when a space is centered around exercise, the ideas that are associated with this concept, and the ties between fitness, eugenics, and the medical model. Ultimately, I decided it was not possible to facilitate fitness practices without contributing, in some way, to the mechanisms that preserve the fitness-industrial complex.

So, I opted out.

I still support people who are curious about their relationship to movement in all contexts, not just practices that include specific exercises or programming.

I am motivated by the idea that we learn through movement, doing new things, and through play, creativity, and curiosity. I believe that we are all entitled to our own experiences and it is not any coach, teacher, facilitator, or guide's responsibility to create any specific experience or body state for someone else.

Can a movement coach or guide find community, financial support, and the energetic bandwidth to create spaces for people to have their own experiences with movement, though? I think so. I'm going to share my approach and story, but I want to be clear. This is my experience. I encourage you to develop your own recipe and come to your own conclusions.

We cannot address fitness or work without considering the embodiment of capitalism. I'm not sure it is possible to escape capitalism in the western world. I imagine that even people in off-grid intentional communities are still impacted by capitalism, from using vehicles produced by these systems of labor to the way capitalism has impacted the very earth we live on.

I think about this a lot when it comes to my own relationship with money and what it means to "do business," to "be successful," and how I engage in relationships with people in exchange for money.

When I owned a movement studio, known as Sweet Momentum Fitness, I was challenged by and ultimately found it impossible to run a financially sustainable business that accessibly served the people it was designed for and to care for the people providing these services. I wanted to keep classes small, financially accessible, and to focus on things like universal design while providing trainers—including myself—a living wage, benefits, paid time off, and education reimbursement. My attempt to successfully hold it all together came at the expense of my own livelihood. I worked over twelve hours a day, often six to seven days a week, and was always grinding toward a goal of cutting back, a goal that never really seemed attainable in reality. Rest became increasingly urgent. I was exhausted, in pain, and didn't have an identity outside my work. I closed the studio knowing I needed to create something else, but not really knowing what that was.

I started with what I'd been noticing about the fitness-industrial complex. It seems like fitness relationships often function to create reliance. It creates a dynamic where someone else knows your body, the movements you need to do, and the way you need to do them more than you. Or sticking to a specific program is the only way to see "results." Many of the people I've worked with in fitness spaces hold the belief that they are not capable of moving safely without input or observation from someone else. This has always bothered me. Movement is inherent to who we are as living beings. If we're entitled to anything, I think freedom of movement is at the top of the list. I'm curious about what conditions encourage this freedom and lead to learning, taking in new information about the world, and being able to try on new interpretations of concepts and experiences. Based on my experiences, I have to conclude that fitness spaces don't create the conditions for this freedom and exploration, even if people manage to attain those experiences.

In *Free to Learn*, Peter Gray details how the human learning process has evolved based on what anthropologists and biologists can surmise.[1] Until fairly recently in the timeline of human development, we learned through playing with one another and in relationship to the outdoors. Children's primary teachers were actually not adults, but one another. Groups of young learners taught each other and learned together. Our education system in general has forgotten that, and many of us never had opportunities to imagine and create growing up, instead having stories and information delivered to us to memorize and act upon.

I dream of movement spaces that hold imagination at their center and encourage it freely. Communities where we are able to play, be curious, and learn together but have our own individual experiences and follow our own individual interpretations and whims. In these spaces, guides and coaches would bring their ideas and suggestions as transparent invitations rather than absolute truths or the only way. Clients would be able to bring their own ideas, desires, and history into a space of collaboration. We can't create these spaces without making our approaches relational rather than transactional.

I move toward these movement spaces that encourage imagination by observing and questioning my own teaching and the way I present my work and ideas. I open myself up to new interpretations of my actions. I ask myself whether I'm creating an environment that is safe and comfortable for me or if I'm facilitating a space that is open to the experiences of everyone involved.

Language here becomes extremely important. I've landed on the terms *guide* and *coach* to describe my role. Words like *invitation, inquiry,* and *intimacy* describe the way I orient myself to the process of working with another person.

I came to the "way of the guide" through nature guide Tam Whiley and later Nadine Mazzola as I participated in a program to become certified as a Nature and Forest Therapy Guide with the Association of Nature and Forest Therapy. A guide works in partnership with the human and more than human worlds (which includes plants, animals and other wildlife, and all the stuff we often think of as "nature"). They do not try to control it. They are not attached to any specific outcome or results; everything is open to interpretation, but they are concerned with the physical safety and well-being of their participants. A guide participates fully with one foot in the liminal space that exists in the session and another in logistics and practicality.

I am a coach because I listen, ask and invite questions, share my experiences, and encourage my clients to gently push up against their edges—which is usually the purpose of our time together.

I engage in the process of inquiry with someone instead of teach them. I am a part of the process, I don't control it, and though these spaces aren't about me, I am a part of them. This feels vulnerable and risky sometimes. I have to be my whole self—including being wrong, not knowing answers to questions, and making mistakes. I know this vulnerability as a sensation in my body as it rises. This is authenticity, intimacy, humanity. Sharing myself this way creates opportunity for someone else to do something similar—or not. It's up to them.

Through this process of inquiry and observation, I work in collaboration with my client to design invitations—explorations meant to turn ideas and questions into embodied experiences that often exist in a moment without a lot of language or interpretation. I rarely write programming, which usually occurs to me as being unavoidably directive and oriented toward specific results or achievements.

I met Olivia Cadence Luxe, a coach and founder of Ground Up Barbell in Philadelphia. She started a gym in her bedroom. I was so inspired. Shortly after, I started seeing clients at my home, in my backyard, and virtually. I quickly learned that a movement space doesn't require the trappings of a built-out facility, and that the people I enjoy working with don't necessarily care about that stuff. I noticed quickly that sessions had a more intimate feeling to them—it seemed like hanging out in the backyard was more useful for most people and myself than meeting at a big open studio was.

Since meeting Olivia, I've connected with a number of other movement people who work out of pop-up tents in their backyard, rent at a low cost from community spaces, or meet people at local parks, out of a friend's garage, and in many different public spaces. This work can happen just about anywhere, not only in gyms or studios. The quality of a practitioner is not determined by the space they practice out of—though that space does speak volumes about who they are and what they value, for better and worse.

Working from my backyard rather than a typical studio environment cut my overhead significantly, allowing me to convert my single-car garage into an open indoor space so I could host sessions inside during Pacific Northwest winters. It also made it possible to finally shift to a 100 percent sliding scale price model with no one turned away for lack of funds. I love sliding scale and bartering when possible. These practices allow me to be cared for by my community, in the ways that they are able to. I find that there is a pretty good balance between the folks who pay low on the scale and the folks who pay in the highest ranges to support my ability to offer sessions this way.

One of my interests is in designing movement spaces that meet the needs of the people using them. I envisioned a space that was more like a living room than a studio. Cozy, comfortable, equally equipped for lounging, rolling around, and a little chaos. I opted for a completely open space with a small loft that would become my office. The walls are buttery yellow, and I decided to mount diffuse lighting panels high on the walls instead of having overhead lighting (lots of laying and looking at the ceiling), or lamps that could get knocked over by accident. There is a sliding glass door in place of the garage door, and a window that opens.

In creating this space, I thought about my clients—the people I was engaging with at the time, and the people I worked with at the gym who liked to move but didn't like fitness and/or being in a fitness space. What did they like? What were we doing together? What would enhance our time together? It had to be a place that would provide the right amount of stimulation for folks who are overwhelmed by sensory information and also for folks who enjoy lots of sensory information. That meant everything in the space had to serve a purpose and be a cohesive part of the design. I decided to stick to earthy colors and exposed wood when possible. Audio quality was a primary focus. I set up a surround sound system using the speakers left over from the studio and set the sound levels in a range that works with a wide variety of music.

Many of my clients enjoy being outdoors but prefer to be inside. I brought in indoor plants and a little handheld water mister, bouquets gathered from plants outside, and a few smooth river rocks from the land around the structure to bring continuity between outside and inside.

I also wanted the space to transform seamlessly during a session based on how folks show up on any given day. Are they going to be on the ground? Will we be doing squats or deadlifts? Are we going to juggle? Are we going to hang out and listen to music? I put rubber, shock absorbing flooring down (horse stall mats from a farm store), and over it giant, lightweight, and thick padded mats designed for cheerleaders, which cover the entire floor but can be rolled up at a moment's notice. I hung a multi-grip pull-up bar so we'd have a place to hang things and hang from. Are we going to be talking about heady concepts and ideas? I brought in some of the books that have inspired me to have on hand as references. What will we be doing? Talking? Lifting something heavy? Listening to music and relaxing? Incorporate a small collection of movement tools inspired by many modalities and the different styles of activities we may be doing. Sensory tiles to walk on, large wooden boxes with high weight capacity that can be used as seating or for movement, bolster-style pillows and blankets, resistance bands, kettlebells, sand bags, drawing supplies, juggling balls, suspension trainers, and tools for gentle self-myofascial release.

I was on an extremely tight budget and opted to do a lot of the labor myself, using the skills I picked up working in theater scene shops in my late teens and early twenties. It was an exhausting two months that brought up so many unfinished feelings that were left over from some of the most challenging times of my life. The process was often fueled by fear, overwhelm, and exhaustion. Along the way, it was safe for it to be happening in exactly the way it was, no matter how uncomfortable it got.

Over the course of the first year, I worried often. Though I was still working with folks I'd known for years and meeting new people pretty regularly, I was worried that people would stop "finding me" eventually because I'd stopped describing myself with buzzwords that were easily searchable online. I can't imagine many people look up "trans competent and affirming embodiment coach." I remembered some of the best advice I'd received during my early training days. Dr. Beckett Cohen, founder of Q Chiropractic here in Portland, shared their process with me: They participate in the activities they enjoy—whether it's concerts, outdoor sports, or other community gatherings, and they share their passion and interest with the people they meet, as it comes up. What a revelation! Go places you like, hang out with the people you vibe with, and share your passions. Again, a shift of perspective orienting away from marketing and networking and toward community and building genuine relationships.

I realized, as with all things in movement, the process of establishing myself as a practitioner, both inside and outside fitness, has happened over the course of my entire career. Relationships and trust are not built via social media ads and a big marketing budget. In relationships founded on intimacy and care, you can go directly to your people and share the news of your transitions, and they will support you because they will know you and what you stand for. Being held by other people throughout this process has been terrifying and deeply rewarding.

Being a community-based movement practitioner is the process of a lifetime. It is never done, only evolving. Once submerged in the fitness-industrial complex, and always stepping in what bell hooks calls the white-supremacist-capitalist-patriarchy, my relationship with the world is forever flavored by a system designed by my ancestors to perpetuate and transfer trauma. My work and my life are a commitment to remembering ways long lost, peeling away the layers of hurt and stifled exuberance. It is a practice of relating, dancing with vulnerability, and pushing gently against my edges over and over again. Reconsidering my interpretation of history and of what I know to be factual. Fucking up, a lot. And listening, listening, listening.

CHAPTER 10

Embracing the Body after Change

DR. MARCIA DERNIE

The words I use to describe myself did not always define me or feel like home. Let this story serve as a reminder that we always have the tools within ourselves to find empowerment, freedom, and joy.

As I child, I spent my free time on the streets. You could find me climbing a tree or roller skating to Eckerd's to buy some candy. Throughout high school and college I played soccer and flag football. I was always moving in that time, whether it was dancing all night at soca parties or running after school at practice. My family had a YMCA group membership that we put to good use. I joined the group fitness classes and ran on the track as I watched the gymnastics kids practice. I was always in awe of the way folks moved their bodies. I enjoyed watching the dads in all their ace wraps and elbow-sleeved gear squeak on the court as much as I did watching little girls in leotards doing flips and landing on foam boxes. This was neither an expensive boutique fitness studio for a certain clientele nor a commercial gym full of individuals so full of self-esteem issues that you had to shower twice to get their insecurities off your skin. Rather, it was a fitness space where I felt safe, where people from my neighborhood were joyfully experiencing movement together. This atmosphere influenced the way I formed my relationship to fitness growing up.

Looking back through a gender-fluid lens, it's funny that I loved all aspects of movement in the gym but still found the weight room to be off-limits. As active as I was, I never stepped foot into a weight room. As much as I adored movement, I never thought strength should be a part of it. At the YMCA, I stuck to the treadmills, bicycles, and ellipticals like all the other girls. My mother always wanted me to be girlier, daintier, and prettier, which meant that strength training was forbidden. It wasn't even a hard boundary or limit in my brain. It was a fact. Girls stay small and cute, while boys get muscles. Even in high school, the weight room was never shared with female athletes. Now as a physical therapist, I realize, wow could I have mitigated the shit out of most of my soccer injuries with a little strength training!

When I graduated high school and moved on to college, I packed all my gym misconceptions with me. The weight section was still an intimidating place. It was smelly, loud, and dark. There were tons of sweaty dudes grunting and looking menacing. Muscle-bound men shouting and dropping dirty metal things. It was not a place for a lady, one where you could get toned or lose weight. Again, I stuck to my fun group fitness classes and on braver days ventured onto the gym floor only to use the cardio equipment.

Sometimes all it takes is one small seed to start a forest, and that small seed wasn't even planted intentionally. In college, I still lived at home and frequented the YMCA. One day leaving a group fitness class I overheard a conversation between a femme trainer in a larger body and her student. She was explaining muscle building and strength to this student. Somehow, I walked by and heard the lines, "Yeah, muscles are muscles! I have tons of fat, but under this is tons of muscle because I lift weights." My knee-deep-in-diet-culture ass walked by this conversation and thought, "Well, what if I didn't have any fat? If I start lifting weights and get muscle, I'll be fine as hell!" After working hard to get rid of my "freshman fifteen," the idea of having muscles became appealing. I'd seen the college teams of women with shredded six-packs and sculpted legs and decided I would love to look like that.

And **BOOM** everything changed. I found a new avenue for movement outside organized sports and group fitness. I went from worried about the shape of my arms to worried about how I could increase my squat numbers. Somehow, once I touched the barbell, I was less concerned with how my body looked and more amazed with what my body could achieve. I was also less afraid of the gym with my high school buddies by my side. I was cushioned and safe in the commercial gym weight rooms, surrounded by my best friend and my future husband at every workout. They softened every misogynist blow that was handed to me, and they lessened the sting of every micro-aggression. Soon, I was a god at the gym. Men would clear the squat racks when I came in, women would ask me for strength advice, and the front desk finally stopped trying to sell me personal training sessions.

Within a year of touching that barbell, I competed in my first powerlifting competition. Back in 2010, the sport was not organized or even close to popular. At the local meet, five women would show up and get to know each other and often become a group of friends. So not only had I found a new avenue, with my first competition, I found my first fitness family. After this meet, I quit the commercial gyms and stuck to working out with strength athletes where I felt celebrated. From there I went on to break Florida state records and compete on national stages at several championships. I traveled across the United States for these competitions and enjoyed pushing my body to its limits. Admittedly, I had traded my obsession for numbers on the scale to numbers on the barbell. That is, until 2015.

In 2015 when I was working my first nine-to-five job out of grad school, renting an overpriced apartment, and newly married to my high school sweetheart, I started experiencing issues related to my invisible illness, which I was unaware of at the time. My body stopped behaving like the body it had been for twenty-five years. It started doing weird things, painful things, unexplained things. It started with waking up with a racing heart. One day I woke up with an impending sense of doom. I headed straight to the ER to be jabbed and interrogated. I feared the worst, but besides my family, nobody else did. The attending physician kept probing for ways that I could have caused this to happen. Was it a panic attack? Drugs? Stress? Other drugs? She couldn't believe that I didn't cause the irregular heart rhythms. She didn't think there was anything else to be investigated. After a night stay, I left with more questions than answers and a six-thousand-dollar bill.

For two years, I had testing from various specialists. I found myself getting my hopes up every time a random or rare disease was mentioned, then disappointed when all my results were normal. It was terrifyingly stressful to hang on to a diagnosis and then have it float away. All the while, struggling to pay the costs associated with all the tests. Now, all the specialists didn't have ideas or tests lined up. Some of these doctors decided to go the gaslighting route instead. "You just have anxiety; try meditation" and "You're young! I'm sure it's fine." Or "Why don't you stop worrying about that and start worrying about having babies?" These all became familiar phases. I continued to push forward despite strange feelings of somnolence, body aches, and menstrual changes. I pushed myself working three jobs, and I pushed myself in powerlifting competitions.

In 2017 I finally made it to the big leagues and was set to compete with the top 10 lifters in the nation for my weight class. The year before, I was real salty about not making the cut for the top 10 primetime competition stage. And even saltier when my body surprised me with heavy fatigue and a menstrual cycle two full weeks early. Needless to say, I went into this 2017 nationals with big "something to prove" energy. I obsessed over my competitors' lifts, programming, techniques, weak points, best lifts, coaches, gym, and **MORE**. I strategically planned which lifts to share on social media and which to keep to myself. I stalked everyone else's media for clues. I planned my weight cut perfectly to meet the weight class limits and packed everything I needed.

Denial is a helluva drug, and it eventually wears off. I left my mother in a hospital room to drive three hours to this national championship. I thought, my mom will be fine and I'll do great! I had no trouble making my weight or getting settled in with a good meal. My body felt well rested and ready to wreck the event. I got dressed and started warming up for the squats. I was in full denial and ready to dominate. But my mom was not fine. And I did not do great. As I racked a warm-up weight, I got a call from my oldest brother. I'm sure he knows what he said, but I can't remember a thing. All I know is that he told me my mom had leukemia. For the rest of the event, I barely connected with my body or the lifts. I missed most of my squat attempts. I think I got my bench attempts. By the end, I was experiencing intense vertigo and feelings of dissociation. I told my coach something wasn't right, and we lowered my deadlift opener to a number I could do with my eyes closed. I made that first and only attempt, then rushed back to the warm-up room to lay on the floor for thirty minutes straight until the all-consuming vertigo feeling passed.

When it did pass, I got up and kept the world-crushing news, rushing thoughts, and disorienting body feelings to myself. I smiled and nodded and took pictures as the event ended and winners were announced. I shook hands and exchanged hugs with pals from the internet who were excited to finally meet IRL. I ignored the curious looks and the presumptions about my performance. And finally, I went home and accepted my circumstance. I had another embarrassingly meager performance on a national stage. It's a huge blow to your ego to be on track to hit a three times bodyweight deadlift to barely staying upright on a national stage. Oh, and yeah, my mom was probably going to die.

My lovely mother battled with leukemia for three solid months. If the week has seven days, I spent six and a half of them taking care of her. Every moment that I spent away from her in the hospital or left her to sleep alone at night at home, I felt guilt. Somehow, I became her only support despite our huge family. I was the one she asked for favors. I was the one she wanted to be cuddled by at night. When we lost her, I lost any semblance of normal left in my body. Because of the stress and loss, my symptoms increased beyond irregular heart rhythms and periods. It was full-on muscle spasms, brain fog, nerve pain, choking and trouble swallowing, tripping over my own ankles, and falling. It was **BAD**. A few months after she was laid to rest, I decided I had to stop pushing and stop running. Despite being broke, I stopped struggling to work at my three jobs and quit two of them. I did not compete after 2017, and my gym sessions were few and far between. I booked more appointments with specialists and started digging yet again.

My loss taught me the fragility of life firsthand. If life can be taken in a day, month, or year, how could I waste any more time?

A Journey to Self-Nourishment

I had to make some decisions in making my time worthwhile. Grief was its own thing. But adjusting to this new body? Embracing the body I lived in? I could work on that.

The first barriers to embracing my body were shame and anguish. I had to let go of the feeling that things were my fault. The feelings that I had to find a magical cure that would fix the problem that is my body. The feelings of anguish over losing the person I used to be. All of these negative trains of thoughts and patterns were weighing me down. I realized later that these feelings were manifestations of internalized ableism. Ableism essentially devalues, dehumanizes, and discriminates against people with disabilities. Disabilities that may be seen or unseen. The idea that the changes in my body were my fault grows from the ableist roots. I truly believed disability to be "bad," and that if I only did "good" things, I wouldn't have any disabilities. The idea that I needed to fix my body, also ableism. There is nothing inherently wrong or broken about disabled people, but that was something I believed before I got sick, so that was something I turned against myself once I did get sick. The intrusive thoughts stemmed from ableist ideals that always existed but had never been relevant enough in my life to warrant thought, exploration, and unpacking.

I grieved over the older version of me and all that was lost. I never took time to acknowledge my humanity or worth. I never took a real moment to think about the changes that have come and gone with my body. I never took a real moment to think ahead to the changes I could still look forward to. I decided that this moment was the only moment that mattered and tethered myself in a corner with no opportunity to be free. Somehow, I realized I needed to reframe these thoughts and patterns to break the cycle. Maybe it was engaging with online communities like Disabled Girls Who Lift, or reading numerous threads on Twitter with the hashtag #NEISvoid,* but somehow, I started to realize something that helped me break the pattern of learned helplessness and dampen the noises of internalized ableism.

This learned helplessness manifested as low self-esteem, feelings of being a failure, avoidance, and low motivation. I held the belief that my body was

---

* "#NEISVoid is a hashtag that No End in Sight host Brianne Benness created in March 2020 to centralize conversations about life with chronic illness and the diagnostic process that were spilling over from this podcast onto Twitter." "What Does #NEISVoid Mean?" No End in Sight, accessed July 15, 2022, https:// noendinsight.co/neisvoid-explained.

worthless no matter what I did because no doctors could diagnose or cure me. I truly thought that no matter how hard I tried, there was nothing I could do to change how my body felt. I ruminated on the notion that my body would always be weak and get weaker, and that this weak, sick body would be a burden to those I love. After months and months of anguish and shame, I had to take a full stop on negative trains of thought. No matter the circumstance or situation, I had to acknowledge I was still a whole person worthy of good things. I was a whole person experiencing a bump in a road that could not alter the construction of my being. It could not change the foundation at the very core of what makes me, me. No person, no diagnosis, no medical problem, no physical injury, not one thing can take that me away from me.

I broke this pattern by reframing my thoughts. At that time, I had my close friends and family, but none of them understood my struggles. I leaned into free online resources from disabled folks for disabled folks. I've never been one for nonfiction, so I didn't pick up any books in particular. But I followed folks on social media, found online communities like Inspire, and read blogs. I explored my thoughts and discussed all the icky negative and dark ideas with my disabled friends. At the time, I had crappy insurance and could not afford the money to spend on therapy, nor the time to go. I was working three jobs and barely getting by. Somehow, I did this mostly on my own.

First, I acknowledged that I felt helpless. Then I battled the persistent thoughts by shifting the perspective. I stopped blaming myself and my body for everything. I ceased a practice of taking situations or conversations personally. And I stopped speaking in absolutes and started giving myself more agency. I pivoted from "a change is happening to us" to "we are working with new changes." I turned away from "a doctor needs to name this problem and give me a solution" to "I need to learn this body and work toward solutions."

I also dug into the ableism that plagued my thoughts. At this point in my fitness journey, I unpacked and put to bed misogyny. I was perfectly fine with taking up space and lifting weights. I began to hate the word *tone* as a descriptor of muscle and encouraged all my femme friends to lift weights. But I did not unpack or even understand ableism. Despite a career in physical therapy with disabled folks, I had the wrong picture of disability. Disability in my mind meant miserable, unemployed, and living in a wheelchair. It meant loneliness and a life of feeling sorry for myself. This is what I saw in some patients and what I chose to perceive for everyone. In my brain I programmed yet another binary: disabled = bad, able-bodied = good. And when I found myself approaching the crossroads of becoming disabled, I couldn't handle it. I broke these patterns with community. Somehow the universe rewarded my Instagram algorithm with chronic illness havers and limb-different women who were lifting and thriving. I connected and vented. I unpacked and settled in. I even started a podcast through one of these connections called Disabled Girls Who Lift.

I learned that disability, like gender, resides on a spectrum of possibility that cannot be narrowly defined. Disability, like gender, is not a concept that can be split into two separate boxes. There's a lot of gray area. Disabilities can be physical (seen or unseen) or mental ones or both. Disabilities can happen before birth, during birth, in adulthood, or all of the above. The same exact disability or illness in one person may present differently in another. The same exact medication or conservative treatment that works for one person is horrible for the next. With that in mind, we can't create narrow expectations for what people can or can't achieve. There is absolutely no way to tidily put disability in a box.

With that, I tackled my intrusive thoughts. I won the battle. I still hold sorrow and pain for the things that could have been while honoring that something is better than nothing. And that something might even be better than what I thought was lost. I realized that bad things won't last forever, and I have the power to change how I think, feel, and move. I took back my control and started helping myself.

I reclaimed my time by hiring and firing doctors as I saw fit. Doctors spent more time gaslighting my concerns than reading my chart? Fired. Doctor told me to "just get over it because we'll never find an answer"? Fired. I reviewed all my medical records and requested changes where doctors deliberately lied. I sent my reviews and reports directly to doctors' offices and filed grievances with insurances. I also reclaimed my power by accepting my body. I may not be able to stop every flare or reduce every symptom, but I realized I can choose how I adapt. I learned to take control of my recovery and healing to make positive changes. I also gave myself grace for "cut and dry" orthopedic injuries, understanding that nothing in this body will ever be simple again. I learned that although everything that happens to my body isn't my fault, I still have control over how I respond.

I responded by setting myself up for success as much as possible. I did not pick up where I left off. I understood that my body lives in "the after" now, not "the before." And the after requires a little more care. When it came to returning to movement, I took my time getting acquainted with a new body. I planned for active recovery with bodyweight and light resistance movements. I gave myself more rest days than exercise days, so I had a full day to assess how my body felt with each re-introduction of movement. I spent weeks trying out different supplements for pain and fatigue to assess their usefulness. I spent months taking notes on my symptoms and the variables that altered them. I paid more attention to sleeping, drinking water, and eating balanced meals. I stopped restrictive diets and focused on intuitive eating. And I began to embrace self-care. I gave myself permission to be stress-free for any given moment of time and nourish myself. I let go of the need for daily productivity, ideas of laziness, and an aversion to rest. As I became reacquainted with my body and movement needs, I was also getting reacquainted with fitness spaces. Many of these commercial gym spaces place the expectation of weight loss and aesthetics, while strength gyms place the expectation of achieving strength at all costs. Big "no pain, no gain" energy. Getting in touch with myself meant getting out of touch with these expectations. It meant not giving a shit about what folks said to me about how I choose to move my body. It also meant learning to discern when not giving a shit meant nodding and smiling, or educating.

Embracing the changes in my body required a few tangles with the mind and a bit of movement. I am not cured of negative feelings or thought, but I am better equipped.

I do want to take this space to elevate my fellow spoonie sisters and women of color. Merely existing is a damn task. Anything more is extra credit. Trust me, of all people, I get that. Thank you for being here, and thank you for giving yourself the space to grow.

And to all, now you know me. You know my story and my struggles. You've always got a helping hand in me.

On the next page, you'll find a handy flowchart to sum the steps I took to embrace my disabled AF body. Run through when you need a quick reminder. It's a tool I wish I had to keep me on track, but since I've already figured it out for me, I might as well give you all a head start.

Embracing the Body After Change

By Dr. Marcia Dernie, PT, DPT (@thatdoc.marcia)

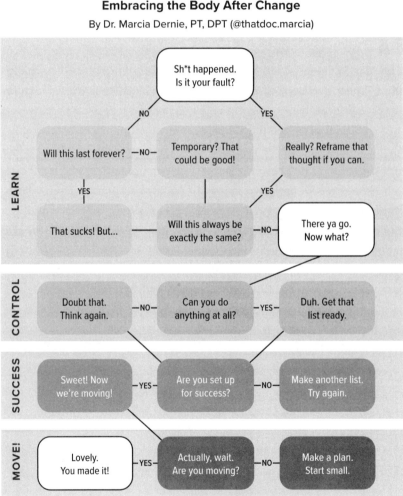

CHAPTER 11

The Body as a Site of Oppression and Freedom

DAMALI FRAISER

Coach Justice Williams asked us an important question during a very powerful panel discussion between Black and white women-identified fitness professionals. He asked, "In what ways have you experienced your body as a site for oppression?" We all agreed in our response, saying, "When have we **NOT** experienced our bodies as a site for oppression?!"

◆

Most folks know me as Coach Damali. They know me from my movement practice and kettlebell training. Training with kettlebells came to me through an unusual path starting with Muay Thai. The art of eight limbs, this is a martial art of kickboxing with elbows and knees from Thailand. Muay Thai was my first rebirth in fitness, but kettlebell training is the first place where I have felt completely comfortable laughing, crying, and just being in my body. Strength training with kettlebells has helped me reconnect within myself in ways that make talking about the oppression in my body necessary and facilitated my healing. You might already be curious on how a Black woman in her forties ended up participating in the national sport of Thailand and then settled into teaching another considered to have originated in ancient Russia.

One reoccurring experience for Black people in Canada, no matter where you live, is to always be asked "Where do you come from?" I was born here on the traditional territory of the Mississaugas of the Credit, the Anishinaabeg, the Chippewa, the Haudenosaunee, and the Wendat peoples, which is now home to many diverse First Nations, Inuit, and Metís peoples. My parents and grandparents were born in the Caribbean. Those are my roots. Canada is where their seeds were planted. For me, a Black Caribbean Canadian woman, my blackness is what people see first.

◆

Loss is a trauma that some can speak on and many others can't. I talk to my students and clients frequently about the process of grief. We are usually talking about wanting your body back or letting go of what you imagined your business or life to be like at a certain age, but my experiences of loss are inextricably tied to one another. They are the places and times when I connected or disconnected from myself and my body in many hard-to-explain ways.

During my baptism, when I was sixteen, I laid a picture of my four-year-old brother at the cross. This was five years after his death but only the beginning of me trying to deal with his loss. Like many, I think this early loss led to coping and numbing with food. There was a pain in my body that I couldn't articulate at a young age, and I filled that with the pleasures of eating. The result was putting on weight and seeing my body not through compassionate eyes of grief but through the lens of something always being fat and therefore something being wrong with me.

Growing up I lived in two households: my mother's house with her partner and their children, and my father's house with his partner and their children on weekends. None of my siblings lived this lifestyle. I was the oldest and the only one who traveled between households. Usually, people are surprised that

I am the eldest of ten siblings because, in a weird way, I have always really functioned as an only child.

My father lived beside a house with a backyard pool. You know the one where you hear the splashing and the music playing on warm summer days. When you don't have a pool as a kid, you often think about how you can get an invite over there to the cool house.

I imagine that my brother felt the same, that he felt hot and it sounded like they have fun over there, so one day he went over. He took all his clothes off and jumped in the pool. He wouldn't have known that side was too deep or that swimming was a skill and not just for fun.

I was with my mother's family when it happened. From what I remember, I was told that my dad found him, tried to do CPR until someone else came, and then they took over until the ambulance arrived. I have children now and can't imagine what that would have been like for him. It stifles my breath and brings tears to my eyes.

They called me and told me what had happened and said my little brother was in a coma. I was eleven and I don't remember how I got to the hospital, but I do remember the hospital room, the smells, the adults around his bed, and the way they parted and made a space for me to get closer. He was so small, and there were so many tubes and pieces of equipment connected to him. He wasn't breathing on his own. He was there that way for over a week. I think it was ten days. Then they said he wasn't coming back and they had to let him go.

His mom had always been a very strong presence for me. I called her Auntie although she was with my dad as long as I could remember. She'd had three children with him and had one more on the way at the time. At the funeral, they escorted me up to say goodbye. It was an open casket, and I struggled long after to erase that picture from my mind while trying to hold on to the memory of him before. I always wondered if she had felt strong sitting there in front of him.

After the reception, they found a toy voice recorder of his at the house. It had a tape, and on it was his voice singing. They were listening to it to remember him. But his voice wasn't the only one on the tape. Mine was there too, and I was singing with him. We were just playing with no knowledge that would be a memory of his voice.

After this time, I lived in only one household. It's not surprising that my father's household was sad and he didn't want to bring me there. They were grieving and I was grieving, but I felt left to grieve alone.

—

As a young Black girl, I never understood how much my body would endure and hold on to. There's no doubt in my mind that I have carried each of these experiences within my body with no real understanding of how to find myself beneath it all.

With immense vulnerability, Margaret K. Bass discusses being a fat Black girl in a fat-hating culture in *Recovering the Black Female Body: Self-Representations by African American Women*:

> Fat Silences. That makes you alone and lonely even when you're nine or ten. The truth of it shames you; you do not tell when people hurt you. You are ashamed to admit that you are fat—ashamed to be fat—so you do not tell unless you find someone who cares and understands.[1]

By the time I was fourteen years old, I was fat at size 12–14. I had already been warned so many times to be prepared because "just look at the size of the women in our family." I was told to "watch what you eat," exercise, and be on a diet in order to prevent the inevitable, that I would be fat, Black, and that would lead to everything awful. I tried SlimFast shakes, which started the trend of skipping meals and eating more salads, because you only need two shakes and one healthy meal to get SlimFast, right? We didn't have much, so the cheaper the better.

I was called chubby, chunky, thick, and curvy and shopped in the women's department starting at age eleven. Being called fat was painful—until it wasn't. Let me explain.

Toward the end high school, I was introduced to rugby, a sport that uses a ball that looks like an American football and running cleats. It was the first team sport I'd ever tried out for, and I dedicated myself to participate in games against other schools. I was a forward, which for those who don't know about rugby, are usually the bigger people. At just over five-feet-five,

I'm definitely not big and tall; I was just big and strong. During this season of my life, I became very active for the first time, so it became the first situation where I lost a lot of weight.

I came to understand what thin privilege felt like. My clothes started falling off my waist. My pants were terribly big, and I'd have to wear belts to hold all my pants up. I wore crop tops for the first time in my life. There are very few pictures of me during this time because I never really reconciled with myself that I was truly thin. I was now playing a sport where I felt immensely powerful, but I was not as small as some of the other athletes.

Being in a primarily white environment in schools, I hadn't really been dating early on. I had crushes on some of the little white boys, but I quickly learned that they didn't like chubby me the same way as the white or non-Black girls. But now I was in high school and experiencing a phenomenon that happens after people lose weight, where suddenly people liked me a lot more. They invited me to parties, they paid attention to me, and girls asked me how I did it. For me, at this point, fitness always began tied with an appeal of getting thinner to improve aesthetics and beauty, which would then result in gaining love and friendship. Being new to this body and this environment, I still didn't fit in with the girls and athletes who had always been popular at school, but getting more attention from Black guys outside school increased. My involvement in fitness and my new athleticism correlated with receiving love.

When a slightly older guy started paying attention to me, it was welcomed. The fact that that experience ended tragically is a common story for many Black women, unfortunately. Young Black women's bodies are often objectified and hypersexualized. He took from me and then left.

Growing up in a mostly Christian environment, I felt I deserved this treatment, this event, because I must have been asking for it by flaunting my newfound physique. I retreated back to eating for comfort and coping with the assault. I began unconsciously putting on weight because it's easier to hide in a fat body than in an appealing, thin one.

I met my husband only two years later, at eighteen years old. We dated for about five years before we got married and had our first daughter. Our lives went into parenting mode. All my focus was on how to take care of this innocent little person who needed everything from me. Following pregnancy, however, I was bombarded with the message of "getting your body back." Moms are tasked with joining fitness groups and trainings in order to recover their pre-pregnancy bodies and lose the baby weight; it's like being a magnet for people to provide unsolicited advice and suggestions on the next diet and exercise program in order to get me back into shape. This was probably a natural thing for me after my childhood days of SlimFast, but I just fell into a continuous stream of diets, Weight Watchers, LA weight loss, looking up Dr. Bernstein, and trying every diet and exercise routine out there, including Beachbody's P90X and Insanity.

It never occurred to me at the time that every step of the way, my daughter was watching me and learning what it was to be a Black woman building a relationship with my body through food and fitness. My initial example of fitness was one of continuously looking to exercise to lose weight, to change my body, and to prove that I didn't have to look like I'd had a baby. I became a working mother. I can remember having many days when I would come home from work and just fall asleep exhausted on the couch with little energy to give back to my little person. Then came baby number two.

I am a survivor of gender-based violence and never felt I could bring that part of myself into the fitness world. I am passionate about the well-being of Black women and see strength radiating from all of us, in the way that our hair twists and curves in countless directions that braided together only persevere and endure. I wanted to protect my daughters, so I went looking for martial arts training to teach them discipline and self-defense through punching and kicking. In that search, I found out I needed to punch and kick things just as much as they did.

A Muay Thai workout provides both aerobic and anaerobic training, usually sixty to ninety minutes, and it will completely deplete you and leave you drenched in sweat. Those first few workouts I thought I would die. I was completely emptied out, and that was exactly the physical exertion I needed to realize I needed more from myself and I was made for more than I had ever realized. How come it couldn't just be fun? I really don't know. The pursuit of thinness is praised in the Muay Thai community. Even if you don't want to compete, the ultimate accomplishment is to demonstrate how Muay Thai could transform a body, and that must include weight loss. I did it. I lost over eighty pounds and dove into competing as an amateur Muay Thai fighter for three years.

At no point during the duration of my fighting career did anyone ever say the weight lost was enough. There was always a lower weight class or smaller body recommended. Additionally, as a lean, muscular Black woman the comments got more aggressive: "That's too much muscle," "You look like a man," and "I like my women softer." Women are never given a break when it comes to our bodies. Women athletes, especially Black women, are often labeled masculine for failing to conform to expectations of cisheteronormative beauty standards, which are generally white femininity.

But the praise was much louder than the insults. Praise started with just a few more smiles when I walked into the gym, then the office. Folks would start to say, "You look great! What are you doing?" Then it would be amplified with, "Your husband must be so happy to get you home tonight." When I would have a dessert, it would be, "You earned that. You look great." I felt seen. I felt welcomed into spaces like never in my life.

I've more than gained back the weight I lost during that time, so it's hard for me to look back on pictures of me from when I was visibly thin and what many would call "toned." Cheekbones and jawline prominent with no double chin in sight. There were a lot of things for me to unpack following this time of my life. I had a real addiction to thin privilege. The compliments and the assumption from many that I was "healthy" because I was lean became everything. After my first knee surgery I gained weight right away. It brings up questions: If I'm not lean, am I not healthy anymore? If I don't get compliments on my body, am I not a hard worker? Am I unworthy of love and respect? If I feel sad and depressed, is it just because I am fat and therefore ugly? A lot of my smiles had questioning eyes both before and after weight loss or weight gain.

There's a specific picture of me that I never shared much after it was taken because, at the time, I was consumed by my stomach rolling over my shorts. I was thirty-four, wife and mother of two, but felt so much shame about a bit of stomach "rolls" (which I can see now as pretty insulting to people in marginalized bodies). All my expectations for my life after weight loss didn't happen exactly the way I thought. I kept all my fat clothes at the back of my closet in case I was "fat" again. I frequently said that a ketchup packet was my "cheat" for the day. I weighed myself morning and night. I called myself a "big girl" because I always had been.

I'm not saying it's wrong to care about how you look—it's my body, and I can do what I want. But what I know now is I totally lacked compassion for myself. I have been pretty lean, and I now would be considered "obese," so where does that leave my fitness now?

I was healthy then but not perfect. And it's also true that I **AM** still healthy and still imperfect. And I am fat. To quote Theodore Isaac Rubin, "For the most part I use the word **FAT** because it tells it like it is. Words like heavy and large and stout are euphemisms, and I feel there is no point in dodging the issue. I like the term **FAT**, and I think other people will like it too once its pejorative connotation is removed."[2]

I learned many things on my journey to be lean. I learned I must understand why I'm engaging in fitness, that I must believe in myself and my own ethic and sweat equity, that I must invest in myself with time and energy, and that I must make sacrifices if I want to prioritize my own journey. But there are things I needed to keep learning. I must be compassionate with myself, invest time not just in my own process but in people I love, **EAT** (food is good!), and add gratitude to every moment and every movement.

I am not happy with everything about my body now, but I am certainly overwhelmed with gratitude for everything it's brought me through. Every time I get a chance to train it's with care and love for my body and joy in the way it makes me feel.

My eldest daughter is a powerlifter. She started at fourteen years old; she was quiet and had to deal with anxiety that really didn't work with team sports. She's deadlifted 300 pounds and benched 150. Some people, when they've seen her lift, have asked me: Powerlifting? How did she find that? Will that stunt her growth? How much does she weigh?

Just like when I started Muay Thai, I was looking for a way to build confidence and encourage an active lifestyle for my daughters. How did she start? I brought my daughter to the gym to discover fitness for herself. There she saw a set of women, of many ages, shapes, and sizes, lifting some heavy weights, and in that moment she learned she could do it too.

For people asking about her size and her growth, I would say, "She wears size 10 ladies' shoes. She is grown!" These questions create this strange thing of being seen and unseen that happens in Black women's bodies all the time. As early as nine or ten years old I can remember the same feeling; my body was changing, but most of the white girls around me were not developing as quickly. That change in my body size made some people treat me like I was older when I was still a child. Sometimes people would ask, "What are they feeding you?" It was as though my body was wrong and people could use fake concern for my health to ask about it.

I am no longer lean. The question about my daughter's weight is telling me that I don't look like anything the fitness industry produces, so how would my daughter land in a sport of power and strength? It's because fitness is for all bodies! You don't have to be super lean to be strong. You do not have to be super small to be strong. You actually don't even have to be big to be strong either.

Guess what? You can advocate for strength at all shapes and sizes. Strength can be internal, external, mental, physical, and spiritual. It is the development of capacity and elasticity; to be able to expand and endure forces and loads means building capacity to love, to empathize, to endure to fight another day. Elasticity is about bending. It's about stretching out to protect the more vulnerable and weaker aspects of yourself or contracting to move out of the way and make space for other things to grow and expand.

I tell people now that kettlebells are for every**BODY** because I believe kettlebells are for every**BODY**. Muay Thai taught me that without a strong foundation your skills will always be ineffective. Although I will always love Muay Thai, my focus is on kettlebells now and the transferability of any sports and movement for everyday life. Not everyone wants to fight or be put in the position to be hit, but everyone has an instinct to move without pain. People want to move without a once-simple task feeling like an enormous effort.

As a woman with children, that became even more important when carrying my newborn in their car seat or picking them up when they fell. Those simple, important tasks were minimized when my priorities were centered on weight loss and my focus was to look like I did before I was pregnant. But I had to ask myself, how did that make any sense when I brought an entire human into the world? Even more, that I needed to have the capacity to navigate this world for both myself and my children.

I came to the realization that I wanted a place where folks and especially women could just **BE**. The only thing consistent in this life is change. Our bodies are constantly changing, our goals change, and our priorities change. So if you are a competitive athlete who wants to see shredded abs and quad separation, great! Do you? There are bells for that! For everyday athletes who want to reduce their use of painkillers or other medications that may only provide temporary relief, I'm here to say, "Awesome! There are bells for that, too!"

What if fitness wasn't about looks? What if health was never a size? What if kettlebells were for every body? These are the questions that I started asking when I founded Lift Off Strength & Wellness in 2018. This space was borne out of my passion for strength training with kettlebells and a growing hunger for place that was more representative of people with bodies like my own and who felt constrained by typical "gym-bro" fitness spaces.

I envision a place where fitness and kettlebells are for every body and connect us joyfully, without shame. The fitness industry has been inextricably tied to weight loss scams, fad diets, body shame, fatphobia, and coaches who think racism can be ignored or eliminated with good intentions.

It doesn't work that way right now. Fitness culture has become a toxic and unwelcoming space for too many, and it is time to unlearn and rebuild fitness in our images. Diet culture teaches us to not only comply with Eurocentric beauty standards of thin and white but also hate any voice that resists those impossible standards.

The fitness industry pushes from all directions toward a singular image of success, to be thinner, slimmer, leaner, anything to separate people from fatness and Blackness. We are diverse people, and we should be seen, heard, and valued just as we are, all while building a stronger and happier life.

Leading with compassion, I teach people how to embrace their strength inside and out with kettlebell training. This takes place alongside healing and finding freedom in their relationship with food and eating. You can come as you are, no prerequisites and no jumping over hurdles. You were made for more, not less, and you are the one who determines what "more" looks like for you.

An important aspect of Lift Off Strength & Wellness is partnerships, including those with Fitness 4 All Bodies. When people enter into work where compassion and empathy are at the forefront of their practice, there is a real vulnerability, and with that comes some painful experiences. In partnership with Fitness 4 All Bodies, Lift Off Strength & Wellness now hosts monthly lunch conversations designated as a healing space for Black and Indigenous fitness professionals. We have also partnered on raising funds to support the Indian Residential School Survivors Society following the uncovering of thousands of unmarked graves at residential schools here in Canada.

Black fitness professionals need a place of belonging. As we create more spaces for our communities, we are still bombarded with endless microaggressions as well as certifications, courses, and professional development that are primarily run by white, cisgender, heterosexual men. We are sought out for Black History Month, asked to work for free, as some diversity, then forgotten. We need a place to share our stories without judgment and where our feelings will be heard and validated.

In 2021 I hosted PAIL Stories, the first panel discussion for Lift Off Strength & Wellness. This panel explored the topic of pregnancy and infant loss (PAIL) from an intersectional lens of the experience of Black women, fat, and trans/non-binary people. Together we can remove stigmas surrounding PAIL and create community healing. The mission of this panel was to support those who experience loss during pregnancy, the loss of a child, pregnancy after loss, and infertility.

We have a lot of opportunities when it comes to educating trainers supporting postpartum people. Some people may assume class and socioeconomic status are strong contributing factors to pregnancy and infant loss; they are, but not for Black women. A Black woman does not have to be poor for her life or her baby's life to be at stake. Black women are four to five times more likely to die during pregnancy and childbirth than white women, regardless of income, education, or lifestyle. Infant mortality rate for Black babies in 2020 was 10.4 deaths per 1,000 live births, compared to a rate of 4.4 white babies per 1,000 live births.[3] All of this grief and loss is held inside our bodies on every level, cellular and spiritual.

As Malcom X said, "The most disrespected person in America is the Black woman. The most unprotected person in America is the Black woman. The most neglected person in America is the Black woman."[4] This is powerful, much needed, and still very unrepresented work; we are still almost always the "only" in so many fitness environments that we are continuously disconnected from ourselves.

Movement has been medicine to my body, reconnecting me to myself with daily practice, providing much needed healing, but that healing also requires a concerted effort to support the greater communities of marginalized people. We need to be free to be fat, to be Black, to be queer, to be disabled, to be all the things within movement.

My fitness experience is an ever-evolving process of learning, unlearning, and learning again. It's learning how my body contains and filters through all these things I experience. I love to lift weights, and there are many benefits including increased bone density, improved heart health, and reduced risk of injury—but that doesn't mean it will benefit everyone in the same way or to the same degree. I think we need to remove all positive connotations to fitness and make fitness a neutral exploration, accepting there will be a spectrum of experiences and that's okay. There will be times when you will dance until you're standing in a pool of sweat and you may feel joyous and light, but there will also be times when you might just go for a walk with your hips aching or your feet hurting. One type of movement may leave you feeling great but require a great deal of recovery time afterward. One type may leave you feeling awful but enable you to walk your child down the aisle on one of the most important days of their life. Both are experiences I consider neutral, but they also bring the opportunity for more life and personal liberation.

I don't think everyone even likes the term "fit"ness anymore, and I'm learning more about that. I'm unlearning the expectations that everyone should be seeking higher "fitness" and "better" health. I want to see fitness create freedom in the ways we can share movement and make movement spaces more accessible to all the beautiful varieties of people across humankind. I want to see fitness as a pure expression of our humanity where compassion leads and joy is close behind. For me, to be present in that moment would be a place where fitness would feel free to be fitness for all bodies.

CHAPTER 12

How My Fatness Helped Me Reclaim My Power and Tell My Story

KANOELANI A. PATTERSON, MSW, LMSW

There was always one question that used to plague the corners of my mind and keep me awake at night. There were times when this question, about who I was and what I could be, would give me so much anxiety that it would reduce me to tears or a full panic attack because the thought of answering such a question meant the possibility of a fate worse than death. I had to do everything I could at the time to be anything but that because to be that meant I would forever be different and I would never fit in. What kind of question would make someone like myself feel such fear and anxiety? Why wasn't it okay to be different and not fit in? I would later find out that not fitting in is exactly the most perfect thing I should strive for, but it took me a long time to come to that very conclusion.

The question that kept coming up for me was, "Is being **FAT** the worst thing you can be?"

Until I truly unraveled how deep my issues with my eating disorder, internalized fatphobia, and white supremacy were, it was not as simple as it seemed. The layers I'd have to dig through would be my undoing—and my remaking. It would be how I realized there was power in my fat body, and power in me, and that I too had a voice.

I was aching to use my voice to uplift marginalized communities, but mostly I was excited to uplift myself from the bondage that internalized fatphobia, white supremacy, and my eating disorder had kept me in. I wanted freedom in my body to live just like people with thin privilege live, unencumbered by the daily violence that fat people had to live through with even the simplest of things. Through answering this question and many more that came up, I learned how to reclaim my power and tell my story, and the more I told my story the more empowered I felt by it myself.

Let's go back to that question: "Is being **FAT** the worst thing you can be?" Some people would automatically reply, "Of course not," and give a host of reasons why, but it is rare to get people's true feelings about fatness. But you see how they really feel about fatness in how they treat fat people.

When I was growing up, I quickly got to see how people felt about fatness because it impacted how they treated me, including my own family. For them, the worst thing their daughter/sister/niece/granddaughter could be was fat. I remember being put on so many nonconsensual diets as a kid. Now I know I never should've been put on any diet because that was the start of my eating disorder behaviors and eventual eating disorder, which I am now in recovery from.

I grew up as a military kid, an Army brat if you will, and we moved to a lot of places including overseas locations. When my father finally retired from the military, we settled in Oklahoma. In those early times I didn't even think about a diet or being put on a diet, but that all changed when my family encountered financial issues and my father had to file for bankruptcy. This meant we had to sell our house and move to another area. Moving isn't a big deal when you're from a military family, but the transition would forever impact my life. I was always a quiet kid, painfully shy, and introverted, and I didn't speak to people unless they spoke to me. From the outside, this may have looked like "this new kid thinks she too good to speak to people" and "she's a snob," which is how the bullying started.

I was always a really smart kid, and school was fairly easy for me. I struggled in subjects here and there, but overall I always loved learning and school, until moving to this new school. Now that I look back, this time in my life is when my anxiety and depression started. It was a combination of the bullying and being a Black girl struggling with perfectionism; this is the impact that white supremacy has on us. It tells us, "You have to be perfect, and if you aren't you will be failing everyone. You will never be good enough."

The bullying got worse, and I used food as a coping mechanism to deal with it. This is when I started to be told I was "fat." I was nine or ten years old at that time, and not knowing what I know now, those statements hurt. Everyone said fat was bad. The bullying turned physical many times, and I hid the scars and anything that looked like someone hurt me. They commented about my body and my hair and my clothes; nothing was ever good enough for these bullies. I never told my parents about the bullying. I internalized it like many of the children I now work with do. But I started hearing similar comments at home from my parents and started to see how people feel about fatness, live and in living color.

On many occasions I was encouraged to skip meals because "You could handle missing a meal or two." My mother would put me on diets and have me "watch what you eat" to drop those unwanted pounds. I tried to make them happy, but to make them happy, I had to be thin. No matter how many straight A's I got, I was not good enough because I was fat and getting fatter every day. With the bullying going on at school, and now home, I could not catch a break, and I could not take it. I would make up that I was sick all the time so I could stay home and skip school. It was pretty believable because I was dealing with what I now know to be undiagnosed asthma and allergies. I was congested and was sickly all the time. This went on and on until I had missed so many days of school that the school now had a problem. I finally just broke down: "I'm not going back to school and you can't make me." We ended up in court over those missed days, and we were referred to mental health services, and that's when all my "secrets" started tumbling out: the bullying, the depression, the anxiety, and the suicidal thoughts/plans.

I ended up homeschooling because I refused to enter the school building ever again. It was really the best thing ever for me, but that didn't stop the fatphobia and anti-fat violence that was inflicted upon me by my own family. Instead, it got worse. I was being watched like a hawk because of my reported suicidality and wouldn't be left home alone. They continued to make comments about my weight and what I was eating. This is when I started to hide food. It was easy to think that leaving school meant the bullying would cease. But it didn't stop because it was happening at home, under the guise of "concern" for my well-being. When I think of concern trolling on social media, I think about my childhood and how this tactic defined my young and adolescent years.

I'm slowly unraveling the part the church played in this, too. Our family was a church-going family when I was growing up, and to this day my father still is. I met so many people there and found a support system; it was a mostly white church with only a few Black, Brown, and Indigenous people here and there.

I never realized how suffocating and uncomfortable church made me until I got older. The church has a way of making everything out to be a "sin," including eating—but mainly the "excess of eating," or gluttony as it is referred to in the Bible. Anti-fatness has no bounds. It can be found everywhere, and the church was not safe from that. I realized later this was related to religious trauma and racial trauma, and the legacy of colonization in church culture. One example shows up as purity culture, which I had my fair share of. It ruined so much of what should have been normal teenage development because purity culture literally shames you for being a normal developing teen with hormones. This is also why I stopped going to church as an adult and will never return. The trauma I am still unpacking from that purity culture, fatphobia, and an inability to address social justice issues like racism and white supremacy is not something I can ever be a part of again.

Being in church basically taught me that unless I was perfect in all ways, I would never be good enough, which further reinforced my self-esteem issues and self-hatred for everything about me that was not "like" everyone else. The thing I never realized at the time was I was never going to be "like" them. I was Black and fat and my life was always going to be different, and that was completely fine. Different didn't mean bad; it meant that I was never going to fit their mold. I was uniquely built to withstand any storm, and I wish I knew then what I know now.

When we talk about eating disorders, usually we imagine thin, white women. But the truth is that many people struggling with eating disorders are Black and fat women like me, or they exist at other intersections of identity and expression beyond femininity, whiteness, and thinness. Those marginalized bodies are so often left out of the movement and, with it, their lived experience isn't shared. I don't think we talk about lived experience enough—the experiences that a person has throughout their lifetime and in their body that include all their intersections.

I was never officially diagnosed with an eating disorder, but I know now through much of my work I had one. Most of the reason I was never officially diagnosed is because of a combination weight bias and medical racism, which I now know was an issue for all my doctors and my own internalized fatphobia. I believed the lies of the white supremacist medical establishment and eating disorder professionals and deferred to the images that showed up all the time in media and in literature: all their patients were white and thin. I was Black and fat. I couldn't have an eating disorder. And I lived in denial for a very long time.

Like I mentioned before, I was put on nonconsensual diets as a child by my parents. I often heard my own father say I could handle to "skip a few meals." So when I was younger, I would do just that. When I was still in public school, I would often not eat lunch. I would go hours without eating and then binge and hide food wrappers. I knew if they were found, I'd be in trouble and I would be "imperfect and the bad child that couldn't control my appetite." I would get headaches and feel faint at times, but I would not tell anyone because it was more important for me to be "thin" than to be well. That alone is scary.

When I got to college, it got worse. I made excuses that I didn't eat because I was just too busy with school and work. I would just eat later and binge and binge and binge, and the cycle restarted the next day. The most ridiculous part is that no one ever asked me if I was okay or why I wasn't eating. There was no concern for my well-being, and I now know that it was because I was fat. In people's minds, whatever I was doing to "lose the weight" was good because, to them, fat is bad. And I never acknowledged it or questioned it as an issue until much later.

When I moved from Oklahoma to Virginia after college, the same habits and issues followed me. I started a "weight loss journey" in 2011 because I still had this obsession with thinness. I would always take whatever nutrition or diet advice I was given by a trainer, which included overexercising, food restriction, fasting, and "cleanses."

This experience of overexercising is why I have a very complicated relationship with cardio to this day. I was obsessed with dance fitness, which entails a lot of pounding on your joints, but it's a helluva lot of fun. I met my best friend there. But I abused it. I would do not just one class but two or three classes per day. It had become a competition; if you did more than one class, you looked like more of a "badass" and more "committed" to health. I lost over 100 pounds and it was all done with a full-blown eating disorder and overexercising. This was acceptable to the people around me. When I took multiple workout classes a day, I received nothing but praise from friends, family, and instructors. "You are so amazing," they would say. Or my favorite: "You are an inspiration." I gag when I get told that now. I wanted to be a good fatty so badly. Well, I didn't want to be fat at all. That was the real issue.

In 2015 I was in a pretty bad car accident. I ended up with cuts and bruises but seemed to be okay at first. Soon I was experiencing nonstop back pain and issues with my sciatic nerve. At this point, it had become debilitating. I saw all the doctors and underwent MRIs and other courses of action. I was told that I needed surgery to fix a fracture. They said that the accident itself didn't cause the fracture, but now that I am thinking about it, I wouldn't be surprised if my eating disorder history and overexercising—when paired with the accident—instigated this fracture.

What I remember the most out of these consultations was the surgeon's insistence that, after surgery, I lose even more weight to take pressure off my joints and back. I now know that so much of what I was being told is nonsense, and findings by anti-diet researchers reveal this to be the case.[1] The surgery was successful, but there were many rules about what activities I could and couldn't perform, meaning I relied on my parents for care. My mom came to stay with me for about a month. I now realize that my inability to allow my own mother to help me with things was my ableism and internalized fatphobia. The idea of being even temporarily disabled was heartbreaking for me. I could not be both fat and disabled. This meant I fought my mom to do things and she yelled at me to rest. I finally let her help me, but it took me a lot of time to allow it. I did not want to be seen as weak or unable to take care of myself. What would people think of me? I went to physical therapy and slowly got to a point where I could return to the gym.

At this time, I was thinking about what the doctor had said: I needed to lose more weight to take pressure off my joints and back. While I was at home rehabbing and resting, I had begun doing my own research and found that a lot of what doctors were saying wasn't exactly right.[2] I learned about Health at Every Size (HAES), which promotes size acceptance, the end of weight discrimination, and lessening the cultural obsession with weight loss and thinness. At the time, I did not even know that I did not have to lose weight or that I was being discriminated against on the basis of my size. I thought I deserved the descrimination I experienced for being fat.

I did more research, reading, and started following different fat activists and creators on Instagram. I learned about fatphobia and I learned how fatphobia and anti-fatness have their roots in white supremacist ideology and that they are intertwined. I learned more about medical racism and weight bias—this was one of my most damning discoveries. I blamed myself for every doctor appointment that didn't go my way because I was fat and the doctors were "just trying to help me" by telling me to lose weight. But when I thought back on all my appointments, no matter what I came in for it was always "lose weight." I received horrible care more often than not and was misdiagnosed often. I am convinced that the reason I went undiagnosed with asthma most of my life was because of weight bias and medical racism.

Then I had a complete and utter mental breakdown, including crying and screaming. I could not do this anymore. I could not go on one more diet and stand on one more scale and feel the shame, humiliation, and self-hate.

I could not bear hating myself for one more minute for something that was normal. Being fat is normal. And it was completely normal for me to be fat and live my life in a fat body. I did not need to punish myself anymore. This process mirrored the five stages of grief: denial, anger, bargaining, depression, and acceptance.

I was in denial for a long time about the impact that anti-fatness had on my life and the pain that I endured because of it at the hands of society and my own self, which was the hardest part for me to accept. Forgiveness played a huge role in this part of healing and eventually accepting being fat in a society that would stop at nothing to make you assimilate. I had to forgive myself for the pain I caused myself because I didn't know differently, because I internalized the anti-fatness I felt from society about me, and I tried to make something "my fault" when in fact nothing was wrong with me. My body was just different. Anger was a big part of my healing, too. I was so angry at the system, myself, and the world for making fat people feel like our bodies were a problem and that we didn't deserve to be treated like human beings deserving of respect or our humanity. This anger pushed me to advocate for myself in ways that I had never done before, and it helped me advocate for others too.

Movement played and has played an essential role in my healing process and has helped me reclaim the power that was stripped from me by white supremacy and anti-fatness. I have always been an athlete in one way or another. Even as a child I played sports until the bullying was so bad I had to stop. I played sports for the church I attended, too. I loved movement. But as I mentioned before, movement had become toxic for me because of my eating disorder, and I had to learn to approach movement differently—especially after surgery.

Once I was cleared by physical therapy, I joined a gym and made up my own workouts with a combination of light cardio and light weight training. Later, I added back in dance fitness, but I made my intentions with myself clear: stop when you need to, and listen to and honor your body. I was not going back to overexercising and obsessing over it. One of the first things I did was get rid of my activity tracker because I would obsess over it; no longer would I punish myself if I didn't burn a certain number of calories or hit a certain step count. Then I got rid of the app I used to track food. **NO MORE,** I decided. I was going to learn to listen to my body. This was so hard, but I wouldn't track one morsel of food because it would just put me down a path that I did not want to go down again.

I worked out this way until 2017 or 2018. Then I discovered CrossFit. I knew going in that their history was not great and that they pushed a specific body type, but I still convinced myself to go. What I found in the location I went to in Alexandria, Virginia, Trident Athletics, was a community of people hell-bent on encouraging people and learning how to learn the movements while also having fun. The community was diverse in body size and race and abilities, which made me feel really comfortable. The coaches there encouraged me to try things I never tried before, which in my head I had as things I couldn't do because "I was **FAT.**" I ended up trying Olympic weight lifting, and I was really good at it. All the coaches said I was coachable and a fast learner.

I moved back to Oklahoma in August 2018 to focus on my mental health, meaning being closer to family and my support system. When I moved back, I decided to focus more on myself and my healing. This included continuing intuitive eating, anti-diet philosophy, and doing my work regarding how fatphobia has impacted me. I decided that I also needed a movement practice that would allow me to show up as I am: fat and Black in a space I felt safe.

The gym I found is one I still go to now: Southwest Barbell Fitness. The community was very diverse in body size, race, and abilities, which made me feel comfortable. I started Olympic weight lifting with a coach, and I had so much fun doing things I never knew were possible for me. I learned to forgive myself for the times I thought I was failing when really things were falling into place for me. I made friends, people who consider me family now, who cheer me on through personal records. I switched to powerlifting in 2019, and that's where I've been ever since regarding fitness.

I think what makes my gym feel safest of all is the way it loves and takes care of its members. As much as we all want to crush our goals and go after records, that is not what is most important to the gym. I have seen that gym support people in their darkest hours, and the way they help people of all ages enjoy fitness is beyond meaningful to me. When I first started, many of the early-morning gym clients were elderly people, and them being older did not mean a thing. They were still able to enjoy fitness regardless of their age. I will also add the way my gym has embraced children has been powerful for me to see. In our community we have a lot of people who have children and bring their children to work out with them and watch. Many of those children who once were watching are now engaging in fitness and even competing in sports, and the whole community has gotten behind these children. It has never been about them losing weight or looking like their favorite pop star. The most important thing in our gym community is that the kids have fun and are kind to everyone.

My goals have changed here and there, but I have some constants that have remained the same:

1. If it's not fun, don't do it.

2. No intentional weight loss, dieting, or restriction.

3. Intuitive eating.

4. Listen to and honor my body.

5. Be kind in words and actions to my body.

6. Be physically strong enough to lift a house. (This last one is all jokes.)

As of 2022, I've competed in one powerlifting meet where my squat was 325 pounds, bench was 181 pounds, and deadlift was 424 pounds. I have done things that the Kanoelani you read about in the beginning of this essay would never have done because white supremacist society and diet culture told her that "a fat girl is not an athlete." I am a proud **FAT** and **BLACK** powerlifter. I am a proud fat and Black social worker. I show up as I am now. I no longer change who I am or assimilate to white supremacist Eurocentric beauty standards just to fit in and in doing so lose my power more and more each day. No, I have reclaimed the power that was stolen from me by taking up space and being unapologetically Black, fat, and outspoken, and by standing in my power.

The best ways that fatness and fitness can intersect in a just and equitable way is by putting people in marginalized bodies at the forefront of this movement. Right now fitness looks thin and white, and there is something seriously wrong with that. Fitness needs to be a safer and more inclusive space for folk in marginalized identities, but to do that it has to first admit it is a problem, which it still has not. The only focus has been on thinness, whiteness, capitalism, and white supremacy, which is the direct problem in the fitness-industrial complex. In the fitness-industrial complex, the main focus for many trainers and fitness influencers is how much money they can make, without regard for these issues and the harm they cause.

These trainers and fitness influencers target folk with their weight loss programs and nutritional plans by telling them that they are not good enough in their current bodies. And this is not always overt; they covertly do it with their marketing through social media and advertisements. If we want the intersections of fatness and fitness to be equitable and just, we have to stop this exploitative and predatory way in which people interact with their clients and consumers.

Throughout my essay I have discussed nonconsensual diets and how I was put on diets without my consent by my parents. I want to discuss with you what role this plays in fitness and the ways that fitness can include safety and consent-based participation. I want to discuss with you first about power dynamics. In the case of my parents, I was a child and they had all the power, so I could not say NO I don't want this diet, because in my mind I did not know what consequences I would have for not "complying."

The same thinking can be easily applied in fitness. Trainers and influencers hold and wield a lot of power, and if those individuals are white and thin . . . **THE MOST POWER.** People see these folks as important, and they see the knowledge that those folks give them as automatic truth without question. The problem when you wield that kind of power is you can find yourself telling outright lies to people to gain their trust. Once those folk trust, you can get them to do anything: start a diet or an exercise routine, and listen to any and all advice you give them regardless of what the client wants and needs.

If you are wielding this type of power, you have great responsibility, as does everyone involved in fitness. You need to be honest and upfront about the services you are providing and your background. You need to ask clients what their goals are and what they want most of all. This is not about **YOU** but about the clients. I've seen many coaches, trainers, and influencers use their clients' "progress" to boost their ego and make them more money through "transformation stories." Stop this immediately. When your clients are signing contracts, you should be getting consent about everything from pictures to the type of training being offered and the goals of the clients. This is also where it is important for you to **STAY IN YOUR LANE**. If you are not a nutritionist, registered dietitian, or the like, you should not be creating meal plans, and I might add you should not be giving advice on food at all. **STAY IN YOUR LANE** and refer out if you need to. This is where people have a lot of issues and cause a lot of problems. If your gyms are offering meal plans or diet plans and you do not have those credentials, you should be saying **NO** to offering them. I am also going to mention if your client specifically does not mention food at all, you should not be overriding their consent by just mentioning changing their "diet." I see this all the time. If they don't mention it, you don't mention it. Giving clients advice they did not ask for can trigger feelings and behavior, and we need to be responsible and accountable for when we go wrong and harm people. I think if those things were up front, it would decrease a lot of harm in fitness spaces.

I didn't reclaim my power and learn to tell my story all in one day. This took years of working on myself internally and holding myself accountable. This also required me to delve into parts of my life that I had long since buried and that were extremely painful, even now, to think about. But to get me to a place that I felt power in myself and in my story, I needed to do that work. It also required me to pay attention to the people around me and the energy I and others bring to situations. I learned more than anything how to set boundaries so I can stand in the fullness of who I am. I learned so much about my relationship with food, too, as you have read. I learned that food is not just "fuel" as many fitness influencers claim. Food is culture, food is love, and food is memories for so many people. Food is connected to happy times of love and celebration with those they care for. I am a big believer that people can find freedom and joy in food and in movement practices. Liberation is what I want more than anything for people like me who have been held in bondage by eating disorders, white supremacy, and other forms of systemic oppression. And liberation and freedom and **FAT JOY** is what we deserve.

CHAPTER 13

Moving from Allyship to Solidarity: The Roles We Each Play in Liberation

REBBY KERN (THEY/THEM)

When Will I Be Seen?

I recently sat with old-time friends in the afternoon sunshine waiting for the chill of winter to dissipate. We reminisced about our childhoods and reflected on our educators in schools. I realized then that my distracted and overly talkative nature—at least that's how I was described by educators with negative marks—was a sign that I had skills for facilitation and community rather than failure in the classroom. What would it have been like if the adults in my life showed up for me by supporting my personality, my learning styles, and my natural empathic convening skills? Instead, the forceful alignment to characteristics of white supremacy, beginning as early as grade school, became an underlying theme of my development.[1] This forced alignment was later reflected in systems of perfection and assimilation to dominant culture that I discovered in yoga, wellness, and fitness practices. I judged my body, my hair, my voice, the amount of weight I lifted, how long I could hold a handstand, and even considered hiding my gender identity.

Liberation arrived when I accepted these traits and skills as part of who I am and a way to connect to the world around me. It helped me recognize that the world wants so much from me, to be used for my talents, rather than fully appreciated for who I am. All I've ever wanted is to be seen and to have enough space to arrive, rest, and remain connected.

As I have struggled with assimilation to dominant culture and meeting the needs of others, I have gathered strength to live authentically and wholly, no matter the circumstance.

This essay will explore a few questions I've asked myself along the way, and I hope that you find connection and reflection as well:

1. At what point did I start to believe that doing what others wanted me to do was the ultimate power-building exercise?

2. Why do I consistently allow myself to fall into the pit of burnout where I lose the trust of my vision and prioritize the needs of others over my own?

3. Am I a catalyst for trans and queer liberation within fitness and wellness? Does my community believe in me? Are they proud of me?

These questions resonate for me in this moment as I write these words and show up in my life over and over again. The underlying thread to each of these questions is my personal liberation.

I'm Rebby Kern, my pronouns are they/them/theirs, and I'm a biracial, Black, nonbinary person. I am hard of hearing, adopted, and am a survivor in so many ways. I center my work and vision in the collective liberation of my community. My work has branched through policy advocacy, anti-oppression work challenging systems and institutions, as well as holding space as a yoga instructor. I'm here to discuss ways that our collective liberation must remain seated in the needs of communities we serve—namely, Black, Indigenous, people of color, transgender, nonbinary, gender-nonconforming, gender-diverse people, and people with disabilities, whose needs are rarely centered by systems in the name of collective liberation.

Supporting trans and queer people must go beyond hanging up rainbow flags during Pride month. Centering Black voices must go beyond using the shortest month of the year to dive deeper into racial justice work. In order to create the shift needed to recenter BIPOC trans and queer communities, we must come together to dismantle systems of oppression. We all have a role to play in this work, and it certainly takes every single one of us. When transgender people of color are centered in this work, we have a new opportunity to bridge the divide of "us" and "them." In Lama Rod Owens's book *Love and Rage*, he reminds us that mindfulness will not undo trauma, racism, or the harms of white supremacy. What it will do is offer healing and liberation and a deep sense of knowing our place in the work.[2]

This essay is my personal experience as a trans queer person of color navigating yoga and wellness, a multi-trillion-dollar industry dominated by thin, white, able-bodied, cisgender women. I unpack when I've misplaced my trust in systems and brands while thinking I was power building. I'll share the ways I've activated to challenge spiritual bypassing and white supremacy while discovering my limits and journey through burnout. My hope as you read this is that you challenge where you, especially those who are white, cisgender, thin, able-bodied people, have ignored exclusionary practices by yoga instructors, studio leadership, and wellness influencers when it has benefitted you. And for those BIPOC queer and trans folks reading, that you find these words as a reminder of your worth, that you no longer place the comfort of others over your needs, and center your practice in liberation and healing. You deserve joy, rest, and celebration.

We've Got to Talk about Allyship

Allyship as a concept has been defined in many ways in a multitude of applications. An ally can be someone who uses their power and privilege to combine resources for shared objectives and outcomes. The term *ally* comes from Latin meaning "to bind together." People show up in social justice efforts to support the greater good through allyship. Michelle Cassandra Johnson authored a book in 2017 called *Skill in Action: Radicalizing Your Yoga Practice to Create a Just World*. In it she explores the direct alignment of yogic philosophy and principles to social justice through a lens of race, gender, ability, and additional social determinants of identity called social location, defining our proximity to power. While people with *proximity to power*, a term Johnson uses to describe the unique and salient intersectional identities of people who have more or less power in certain social contexts,[3] are useful to build collective power, it's important to realize that allyship is more than a starting point for critical social change.

There is something to be cautious of, particularly for cisgender, white, straight allies: optical or performative allyship, prioritization of comfort and fear. Allyship tends to happen from a space of comfort, particularly for those who have a closer proximity to power. Allies, holding access to power, privilege, and resources, name their allyship and find ways to benefit from their allyship, while under-resourced and underrepresented communities remain in great need.

Brands we all come to know and love tend to change their logos to include the vibrant colors of the rainbow during June, LGBTQ+ Pride Month, even profiting off rainbow apparel and products. This is known as "rainbow capitalism" or "pink capitalism," which is a term to describe the way companies incorporate LGBTQ+ identities while often still prioritizing Western, white, and affluent intersections. The biggest concern with rainbow capitalism is that it reflects the impermanence of allyship, ignoring deep relationship development and power building among the highest needs for transgender and queer people, namely houselessness, anti-transgender violence, employment and housing discrimination, and access to healthcare and gender-affirming care. This style of allyship checks a box saying to the public that "we are inclusive" while profiting off the harms and systemic marginalization of LGBTQ+ people.

Target has publicly spoken up in favor of LGBTQ+ policy including marriage equality, which passed in 2015, the Equality Act, and challenging anti-transgender policy at the local level by committing $20 million toward inclusive store restrooms starting in 2016.[4] Target has even made decisions to create gender equity in their toy sections by removing "boys'" and "girls'" sections in the toy aisles. Target has become an active ally to the LGBTQ+ community by using its power and resources, including buying power and partnership, to show up for queer and trans people.

However, queer allyship wasn't always a critical focus of this corporate entity. In 2010 Target was centered in a PR nightmare following their financial support to MN Forward, funneling those funds to an anti-LGBTQ candidate, Tom Emmer, the Republican candidate for governor who fought against marriage equality in 2007 during his time as a Minnesota House representative.

Something to consider about these allyship efforts is that Target is redistributing funding to LGBTQ+ serving organizations including GLSEN and the Human Rights Campaign. Target has a standing relationship with GLSEN, the gay, lesbian, straight, education network, donating $100,000 from #TakePride in 2021, adding up to over $1 million back to this education organization.

From an interpersonal lens, performative allyship and activism are deeply present on a personal level, as well as on social media. People living in privilege, particularly white, cisgender, straight, able-bodied people, describe their support and allyship of BIPOC, Asian American and Pacific Islander, queer, transgender, disabled, Muslim, neurodivergent people in limiting ways, sometimes only on social media, but not in action or deed. There's even signs of "virtual signaling" on dating app profiles, where people include buzzwords like "#BLM" or a series of fist emojis, in tone order, almost always starting with white skin tones. Those Instagram and Bumble profiles don't go deep enough to reveal how an individual is centering their allyship in active solidarity, learning and unlearning what they know about communities facing systemic harms.

On June 2, 2020, during the racial justice uprising following the murder of George Floyd, Instagram witnessed "Blackout Tuesday," where users posted a black square to show awareness of police brutality and the murders of George Floyd, Ahmaud Arbery, and Breonna Taylor. Blackout Tuesday began as an effort from the music industry, #TheShowMustBePaused, a brainchild of two Black women, Jamila Thomas and Brianna Agyemang, in music marketing.[5]

This effort morphed into what 14.6 million people participated in as a wave of black squares and silence on Instagram.[6] While social media is important for awareness and offering participation in social change, the movement, the revolution, is not taking place on Instagram.[7] Posting photos at direct action marches, wearing Black Lives Matter t-shirts, does not define a person's activism, and often it can misrepresent allyship. Digital activism has limitations and is simply not enough to fight for the liberation of Black, brown, trans, and queer people. We must continue to take action through solidarity.

Give Up Allyship: Shift into Solidarity and Co-conspiracy

The work of solidarity is to go beyond allyship and instead root in the work as an accomplice and co-conspirator. Alicia Garza, one of the co-founders of the Black Lives Matter movement, describes the need to give up allyship to move toward co-conspiracy. "Co-conspiracy is about what we do in action, not just in language," says Garza, "It is about moving through guilt and shame and recognizing that we did not create none of this stuff. And so, what we are taking responsibility for is the power that we hold to transform our conditions."[8]

In doing anti-oppression work, the biggest fear in white allies is the fear of getting it wrong. This fear keeps people from taking risks. Robin DiAngelo writes an entire book on this topic, *White Fragility*, describing the ways fear of getting it wrong and alignment to perfectionism deeply block people from being effective, empathetic advocates.[9]

An accomplice has an active, consistent practice of unlearning where a person in a position of privilege and power seeks to operate in solidarity with a marginalized group. A co-conspirator takes an active role in dismantling structures that oppress an individual or group; forfeits or leverages power, privilege to transform our societal conditions; takes responsibility for the power that we hold to transform our conditions.

The choice is up to each person to determine the amount of work and discomfort they are willing experience and to find a willingness to use your privilege as an opportunity to support someone or a group of people. This is where meaningful change can begin to happen and dominant culture begins to lose out on the cycle of socialization, a model by Dr. Bobbie Harro that illustrates the specific ways systems reinforce bias to control power and generate punishments and reward for those closer to, or further away from respectively, power and control.[10]

As you explore this essay, deeply consider the ways you are showing up in your allyship and/or co-conspiracy.

There's No Place for You Here

While in college, sitting under the Southern California sun, I came into my own as an activist, advocate, and creator. Now, sure, I am a veteran Associated Student Body kid, where I learned Robert's Rules of Order, gained relationships with local government officials, and learned how to put together a homecoming assembly on a shoestring budget. What I didn't know was that I was becoming who I was destined to be. I was slowly putting the pieces together that my voice has the power to move mountains when paired with resources, active solidarity, and a vision of liberation.

My campus was covered in palm trees and dense green grass, sprinkled with afternoon picnics elevated by laughter. Most days I trekked from the base of campus, where the Matheson Theater held my stage writing and performing joys, to the top of campus, where I found home in the art studio, creating expressions from what my words couldn't convey. Other days, I woke up before the sun to run laps with fellow athletes and watched the setting sun on the tennis courts, where I sharpened my backhands and side steps. My friendships developed in these sanctuaries, where I held the joys, pains, celebrations, and secrets of my peers, many of whom came out to me over time, sharing their queer identities with me. Though we sat on a liberal arts campus, we hid many parts of who we were because of the religious affiliation of the school and the overt denial of equal access to community and even to faith because of who we love or our gender.

We eventually came together to continue the work of years prior to start a Gay Straight Alliance (GSA) chapter, or more commonly known today as

Genders and Sexualities Alliance. This was a place where out LGBTQ students could find solace and where allies could show up in support at the intersections of identity and faith. I was a sophomore and had been elected to the student government as the social vice president (take that to all teachers who said I was too social!). I believed that my social power as a chair in a student governing body, along with student power and the support of professors on campus, could push us to finally reach full acceptance, inclusion, and equity as dues-paying students. After submitting the complete paperwork to become a campus organization, I received an email from the Student Life office. The pit of my stomach fell to the floor. My eyes swelled up with tears. Heat rushed to my face. We were met with the Foundational Beliefs of the affiliated church of the school, which, like many faith-based schools, names that there is little space for LGBTQ communities, simply because the Bible says so.

At that moment I took everything I knew about organizing and, well, basically made a whole scene. The local media got involved as I published my exposé for the city to read and hosted a multi-campus event to bring awareness to the event, featuring the incredible J Mase III, a Black, Trans, queer poet and educator based in Seattle by way of Philly.* The student life department quickly called me in, and I wasn't backing down. We were pushed to the side by the place we called home, where we invested in thirty years of debt, where we found community and connection. We weren't taking no for an answer. While organizing our GSA, I was connected with leaders from sibling campuses across the country who were facing similar pushback and limitations. We later came together to start a national nonprofit that provided funding for collegiate campus groups serving LGBTQ students who were denied support and finances from their schools.

All of this to say, it took over ten years for the school to charter the club as officially unofficially as they can, under the department of psychology. Some change certainly takes time, and this was a small celebration, with hundreds of baby steps, all while staying true to who we are and demanding what we know we deserve.

---

* If you don't already follow J Mase, what are you waiting for? @jmaseiii, https://jmaseiii.com/

This level of activism took me down my path of LGBTQ policy work, moving me from Southern California to North Carolina, a place steeped with white supremacy, old white generational wealth, and vibrant rural communities often placed in the center of environmental racism. I found my voice working for a national nonprofit working with college campuses and universities to advocate for equity and inclusion for safer, more welcoming school environments.

This is important to my story because I didn't know when I started my journey that I would be in this seat today, in my power as a convener and activator. This work is more than fighting for what I know is right. It's about my livelihood as a biracial trans queer person in the South, and the liberation of my community. When my community is liberated, I become liberated. That my existence in a room has the potential to change culture and practices, can bring awareness and challenge, and unfortunately, can also be the source of my harm. So I walk boldly and lead with compassion. And I bring my people with me."

Coming Home to Yoga

My first year of recovery was 2011—it was also the first year I played my P90X yoga disc, the one I mistook as a day-off disc, and discovered what I had been missing. I'm not saying P90X was the end-all be-all of yoga; I am saying it was my first exposure and socialization of yoga. I was able to be in my mind and body without wanting to run, which is why I had turned to substances for such a long time to cope with my childhood trauma, religious trauma, and the pains of my ongoing coming-out journey. After I moved to Charlotte, a pal in recovery invited me to go to a yoga class with her.

It was my first time at the studio, which would eventually become my home studio and workplace, and when I entered the front lobby, I was greeted by bright orange and purple walls and it seemed like a fitting place for me to explore yoga asana. The hallway entrance was adorned with a rainbow flag that read the word **PEACE**. I felt like I had found myself reflected on these walls, full of inspiration and curiosity.

When I approached the front desk, I was greeted warmly and was asked to check in for class. It was my first time at the studio, so the front desk worker had to set up my account. I was asked for my driver's license to capture my basic information. This was when my body became tight, my palms started to sweat, and I was unsure of the experience I was heading into. I hesitantly grabbed my driver's license and handed it to the staff, knowing that my name didn't match what was on my driver's license, nor did my gender. I had no idea what fields this person was going to fill out for me or how it would reflect when I would sign up for a class in the future.

Fear in fitness and wellness spaces for trans and queer people, especially for Black and brown trans and queer people, is common and impossible to fully describe. I've heard it described as shrinking or making oneself small. It's bearing the discomfort without speaking up. It's accepting microaggressions, because why would this space be any different than the rest of the world?

This wasn't my first experience with cisheteronormativity by any means, though it stung particularly hard after finding affirmation in my workplace and community. *Cisheteronormativity* is a term that describes the prioritization and assumption of gender identity as cisgender and sexual orientation as heterosexual. Simply put, it's the assumption that everyone is straight and everyone is cisgender. The assumption met with access to social power creates unique dynamics for those who are transgender, genderqueer, gay, lesbian, and all expressions outside being straight and cisgender. People whose identities are constantly challenged by status quo and dominant culture will inherently face barriers to entry—barriers that white, thin, cisgender, able-bodied, heterosexual people with access to resources do not typically have to experience or consider.

I practiced at this studio for about a year before finding a strong stride in my personal practice. In spring 2018 I was approached by the LGBTQ nonprofit I was working for to receive a scholarship for a 200-hour yoga teacher training. The owner of the studio I had been practicing at happened to be a major donor for the same nonprofit I was working for. It only took a few days for me to accept the nomination, navigate the scholarship application, interview with the leadership team, and receive an acceptance letter to be part of the next cohort of teachers.

The first day of yoga teacher training I looked around the room as my twenty-six kula, or community, members entered one by one to see how many BIPOC people were joining me. A total of three. This contributed to my chosen silence in our white-washed ableist teaching of fifty-five poses under the Baptiste methodology. The teaching team for this training were exclusively white, which is not unique to yoga culture. I won't share much about my yoga teacher training, aside from the truth that we didn't learn Sanskrit or the historical, ancestral roots of yoga; we didn't learn about the eight limbs of yoga, or even energetic lines of poses. We learned, however, point-to-point cues to speak to our students, the Baptiste methodology including root down to rise up. We held frog pose for thirty minutes and practiced in 97 degrees for hours on end during training weekends. All of this to say, I knew very little about yoga when I became a certified teacher.

After my training, I came out to the teaching team and my colleagues about my gender identity. The room became small, and my body lit on fire. I was unsure how people would respond or if I would still be accepted. The immediate response was warm and welcoming. As a scholarship recipient, I was later given an opportunity to be mentored in my teaching by the studio manager on a weekly basis, and soon was teaching a well-attended, prime time class. It felt like overnight I had gone from hoping I would see more people like myself teaching at the studio to then being that very person myself. I was the first nonbinary biracial teacher at the studio, albeit the only. There were a handful of queer teaching staff and an even smaller representation of BIPOC teaching staff. The reality was that no one knew what it meant to have a trans person on staff, how to use gender-inclusive language, especially nonbinary pronouns, or what it meant for the studio and its historically gendered practices.

My studio was willing to have a representation of diversity on their team but were not yet ready to dismantle the internal practices that created barriers to my access in the first place. It was the first time I started sharing my experiences as a person newer to their yoga journey navigating an information system that required me to mark male or female, without deeper representation of who I really am. What it feels like to experience gender bias live in class, by teachers with hundreds of hours of certifications, leading people of all bodies in their journey. And what it feels like when yoga students and teachers say that white supremacy and racism have nothing to do with yoga.

We Can't Ignore What's outside That Door

On September 20, 2016, Keith Lamont Scott, a forty-three-year-old Black man in Charlotte, North Carolina, was shot and killed by a Charlotte-Mecklenburg Police Department officer. CMPD, like many police departments in the US, has been challenged for their use of brute and lethal force and bias in making arrests, specifically against Black and brown men. The city erupted with direct action, sending North Carolinians to the streets demanding justice for Keith Lamont Scott and accountability from the police department.

White allies often assume and argue that police brutality has nothing to do with yoga and conversations on racial justice don't belong in the yoga studio. This opinion especially comes from those who are not directly impacted by fear of police, deportation, incarceration, and violent threats to basic human rights. These ideals reflect toxic positivity and spiritual bypassing.

Toxic positivity is the practice of dismissing emotions labeled as negative, like sadness, anger, and stress, and being met with false reassurance.[12] I'd encourage you to play toxic positivity bingo the next time you enter into a yoga studio retail section. I would bet that you'd find t-shirts, hats, and decor that read "good vibes only," "Namastay in bed," or "spiritual gangster." Yoga culture has become diluted to "good vibes only" and ideals of toxic positivity. There is a deep fear of conflict, which reinforces white supremacy characteristics in yoga and beyond, creating avoidance, neutrality, and spiritual bypassing.

Spiritual bypassing describes the active avoidance of pain and discomfort and often is sourced from the lens of the privileged. "The notion that spiritual healers and leaders were never involved in politics and took a passive stance on the political issues of their time is not just an unfounded assumption, it goes against the very examples they lived."[13] To ignore the pain and harms of communities of color and teach to "release all the bad with your next exhale" is deeply irresponsible. Yoga and fitness instructors need to be mindful space holders, knowing that trauma, grief, alongside joy and pain, happen simultaneously. Yoga cannot undo any of that pain; it is a tool to be present with it.

Cultural appropriation is the practice of a dominant culture taking something from another culture without providing context or acknowledgement of history.[14] In the 1960s, Hatha yoga was becoming more widely known and popular in the US.[15] Quickly, yoga became an asset of men's body building, particularly of white cisgender men. Fitness magazines from the '60s to the late '90s nearly exclusively celebrated yoga through body building as studios opened from coast to coast, quickly turning into a popular fitness activity. With the rise of fitness and power yoga in the West came the loss of ancient Southeast Asian culture, tradition, and spiritual embodiment of yoga. Westerners chose to pick up the physical asana while leaving behind the spiritual principles and tools. To claim that the Western origins of yoga were not culturally appropriative or limited to patriarchal systems is a blatant lie.

The yoga communities in the West were still unwilling to talk about race, impact, and social justice on the mat. Studios, who were actively benefiting from prioritizing whiteness and "good vibes only" in yoga classes, were and are dismissing the reality of the world outside the doors.

Hitting My Stride

I suddenly found myself in the seat of a teacher, holding a newfound access to power within yoga and wellness. I had a global brand backing me and supporting my work. My classes were being featured across the city, and I was even getting booked for corporate classes with Microsoft, Twitter, and Duke Energy. I felt alive. I felt seen. I was ready.

I became a Lululemon ambassador in 2019. My yoga teaching career was still fresh and new, and being a part of a global brand felt like I was entering into my stride. Sitting down at the table at Optimist Hall with my store managers, I raised the question of how my full self would be seen and upheld at Lululemon. Our conversation continued, and I was assured that who I am is exactly why Lululemon wanted me to become an ambassador. I am deeply involved in my Charlotte local community, and as a non-binary trans person of color I represented a piece of community that reflects fitness, wellness, and larger parts of understanding the South.

People around me started to trust my work. Mentors encouraged me to follow my heart in my activism for BIPOC trans and queer communities and generating workshops and learning offerings for the yoga community. As I moved into full-time teaching, I took the upgrade and developed content focused on the liberation of BIPOC, transgender, queer, fat, and disabled people within yoga and wellness. It was clear that this content needed to begin as foundational learning. Many of the cisgender straight white thin students who took my sessions shared it was their first time engaging in content at this level. That they were ashamed of the misconceptions and ideals they were given as kids, and some still acted on those biases presently. To give people the space to unpack these realities was crucial in order to create freedom and understanding.

I delivered my workshop Race, Gender & Bias for the first time in December 2018 to a small group of students in the smallest room at my studio. This became my cornerstone workshop chock-full of foundational concepts geared toward allies who were interested in shifting to a lens of solidarity and co-conspiracy. A few co-teachers attended, parents and their adult or adolescent kids attended, and even my best friends. The session was full of laughter, tears, and "a-ha!" moments. It was the first time I truly witnessed my capacity to change the culture of yoga—even if it meant starting small.

As I was setting up for the session, I recognized that something was missing. If I was on a journey with people who absorb culture as yoga students and yoga teachers, who else do we need to make real change? The people in power at the studio, the leadership team.

During the preparation for the session, I was asked to meet with the marketing team to take photos, prepare social graphics, and create blurbs for promotion and sign-ups. My content was poked and prodded, questioned and revised. But I was surrounded by white cisgender people giving me feedback on content to challenge the status quo in every way. I was encouraged to create digestible one-liners and soften the edges of the module, so as to not turn people away or make people uncomfortable (white fragility at its finest). My biggest fear was that I wouldn't be able to lead this work at the place I called home. That I would be too loud and ask for too much. That I would somehow mess things up for more teachers of color to challenge white supremacy and transphobia. So I followed suit the best I could while remaining true to who I am.

On the day of the session, none of the leadership team attended. No one who made decisions about the marketing of my content attended. Even though this was the first workshop of its kind at the studio, neither the studio manager nor the owner attended. It was devastating. I was willing to do the work for the studio without receiving the utmost top-level-down support for the collective vision for the studio. I was creating a vision for a studio who maybe didn't want that mission and maybe wasn't willing to do the work.

This was the greatest lesson I had to learn. I was still prioritizing the comfort of privileged communities before my own needs. I was willing to do emotional labor for people to still have enough power to disregard me at the end of the day. It was the beginning of my burnout.

Here I found myself assimilating to status quo for the comfort of fragile white folks leading a studio community. I started to prioritize this comfort more so because now I had more at stake. My teaching job was on the line as a cherished mentee and scholarship recipient from the yoga studio's owner, a million-dollar donor for the organization I was working for during the day.

PHEW! This was a lot to take in. And this was the milestone that sent me on a spiral to deepen into the learning of allies who were interested in solidarity but unsure of how to get there.

The World Went Virtual

I had wrapped up my first national program when the COVID-19 pandemic became known to the US and widespread panic took hold of the world. It was March 13, 2020, and I was in a weekend immersion for Yoga 12-Step Recovery. While we were learning about the connections between yoga philosophy and the science of addiction in support of healing, the world began to shut down as we were inside those bright orange walls. By the time we were dismissed on the last day, the studio canceled all its classes, my schedule at work dissipated, and business left and right closed their doors. Quarantine kicked in and our worlds changed.

Variant after variant hit the US, and the way we practiced yoga shifted. We were online, we gave up our ideals of hands-on assists, and we learned to practice with masks.

My new routine included getting up around 7 a.m., doing admin work for my business until about 10 a.m., logging in to Equality NC, and taking work meetings while I went for walks. Of course, puzzles and binge-worthy television were part of my quarantine. In the evenings, I taught live yoga classes online and, on the weekends, I found time to get outside and soak up the smells of spring.

It was a morning, like many others I've grown accustomed to. Or so I thought. This late May morning included the news of a Minneapolis man, Mr. George Perry Floyd Jr., brutally murdered by Minneapolis police. I vividly remember the murders of Trayvon Martin, Sandra Bland, Eric Garner, Michael Brown and the uprising in Ferguson, Freddie Gray, and Keith Lamont Scott. I can still hear the chants "I can't breathe" after Eric Garner was suffocated by police. This one was different. This murder was preventable in every way. This time the world watched a white police officer kneel on the neck of Mr. Floyd for nine minutes and twenty-nine seconds, longer than the originally stated eight minutes and forty-six seconds. The world was home and still enough to watch. There was no running from this. No one could bypass the realities of violence at this level. There was no walking back from naming the longstanding racist practices of systems and institutions. This murder only more deeply illuminated the inequities, the bias, and the protection of dominant culture.

Still, I had been asked, "What does this have to do with yoga?"

Before I could address my own emotions from the murder of Mr. Floyd, my Race, Gender & Bias module was already slated to go live online June 2. I would have been overjoyed if thirty people attended, with this being my first virtual iteration of the content. I was not prepared for what came next.

Overnight, my online session hit seventy-five attendees—it sold out! I kept refreshing my page to see if there was an error. I saw names on the list of students of mine, teachers in the community, not only in Charlotte, but across the world. People dialed in from the UK and Australia. I started a wait-list, and hundreds of people signed up. So I set up a session the following week—which immediately sold out. Before I knew it, I had an admin team of support, volunteers helping me write emails, oversee registrations and logistics, handle payments, and offer emotional support to me as I facilitated back-to-back sessions. I did all this from my living room.

What struck me the most was seeing the names of the studio leaders from my home studio, some of whom were taking the session for the first time. Others had attended the in-person sessions at local studios. I found myself in tears after most workshops, unraveling after holding myself together listening to people discover their bias for the first time, or sharing how they don't feel comfortable sharing facilities with trans people, or how using they/them pronouns just doesn't feel grammatically correct.

It took the impact of nine minutes and twenty-nine seconds to change their minds. How many more would have to die for me to be heard? How many more trans women in the city of Charlotte would need to be murdered until they were heard? How long?

No One Enjoys Being Hushed

My workshops were shared across communities where business owners, studio leaders, yoga teachers, and activists arrived to make commitments toward inclusion in their workspaces. I received accolades, and my consulting work increased. Before I knew it the Rebby Kern Yoga team grew to include two rockstar employees to help hold capacity for the growing requests.

My local Lululemon team members attended my session, which helped open up new conversations at the store level on guest engagement. Lululemon stores historically have been split into "women's" and "men's" sections, so much so that apparel for men became branded as "Lululemon men." With these longstanding practices, not only in wellness but in consumer spaces broadly, the work is rooted in challenging gender stereotypes, social conditioning, and reinforcement of gender norms within retail.

I was brought on as a Lululemon ambassador to represent a community of people who are deeply underrepresented in wellness, yoga, and fitness.

My biracial identity, my transgender identity, my queerness, my body, my disability, and the parts of who I am that people would never know at first glance, don't always "fit" when I compare myself to the mannequins in the storefront or the models on the homepages of the website.

I was made aware, however, of a gender-neutral line of apparel. This was something I got lit up about. I would be able to choose apparel that not only defeats the concept that I have to wear skin-tight leggings and a thin tank top to practice yoga, but also a line of clothing which is not determined by how my body needs to be perceived. Clothing that I don't have to experience gender dysphoria in or have to be misgendered while exploring that "section" of the store. It saddens me to say that this line was "lab," which means it was not available in all stores. I actually never got to wear the gender-inclusive line. It was not available at my store, and it was not available for me to purchase. So for the past years of my ambassadorship, I had to barter with myself on the clothing I wanted to show up in. I discovered high-neck compression tops that fit so much like binders. And I also found clothing that worked with my body in movement, including a range of fabrics I fell in love with. Now, this isn't about the clothing. *It's about being invited into a community of wellness because of my identities, while my identities were not valued and honored up front.*

During my onboarding process, I reviewed every contract, expectation, agreement, and product detail with my management team. As ambassadors we are limited to only shop within our gender—this rule is likely because ambassador discounts can quickly be abused and used to shop for other people, which is not allowed. I find comfort in clothing all over the store and asked if I would be limited to "choose a gender" to operate within for my ambassadorship. Likely, they never had to think of that. They didn't consider how this "rule" would land on me as the first nonbinary ambassador for the team. We agreed that I would not be limited to a single gender, nor would I have to decide which gender to shop. The overview was so gender-specific, and I became nervous about what I had signed up for.

My experience in the store was needing to teach my team about who I am. The space was not ready for me. They didn't know how to honor my needs. I was clearly the first of my intersections to hold this space. What that meant for me was that I wasn't able to enjoy my ambassadorship.

After supporting the education of my team, there were opportunities to support leadership team training and conversations where I certainly was compensated for my time, energy, and emotional labor. Managers of managers caught word of my work and started requesting more information about booking me for other events.

The curiosity and commitment coming from my Lululemon store and beyond helped me believe that a global brand could have the capacity to make radical change to wellness. The internal teams were engaging globally with conversations on racism, sexism, solidarity, and body size, going deeper with hiring processes so that Lululemon staff and educators reflected the diversity of guests and of all people who access wellness, and so that no other ambassador would ever have to question if they have a place on the team if they are transgender or gender nonconforming.

Oftentimes, I've been asked in regular conversation, "Well, what should we do about our bathrooms to be more inclusive?" Or, "Do you think transgender people feel safe here?" Or, even hearing from cisgender white allies, "I want to open a space for BIPOC people to lead classes and hold space." Now, hear me out. I do believe in the redistribution of white wealth to benefit communities of color and those who are underserved. What I don't believe in are allies who are deciding what people need.

Using pronouns isn't about memorizing my pronouns. It's about unlearning the gender bias and stereotypes we've grown up with to drop assumptions of people up front, to witness that gender is a universe and does not truly function in separate parts of a store.

An invitation came across my desk to join the Lululemon digital sweatlife. I was asked to be a facilitator for a conversation crafted around my race, gender, and bias work, to be in front of my peers and proudly say "here I am" and this is what I am up to in the world. I quickly agreed and started the process of meeting the team, reviewing content, and planning day-of logistics.

In the midst of that planning, one of my regional managers let me know my work was going to be featured on the Lululemon global Instagram page @Lululemon. Me?! My work? I wasn't running Race, Gender & Bias in the upcoming weeks but was running a new module called Decolonizing Gender to share histories of gender-diverse communities, challenge gender stereotypes, and resist gender practices within consumerism and capitalism. The post was passed along teams for approval, and on September 2, 2020, my post went live as part of Lululemon's "5 to Follow."

Within hours, I noticed my follow count increase on Instagram. By the end of the day, I was informed that the post was getting negative feedback and the comments were having to be monitored and eventually turned off altogether. Within days, I was on the line with my local team, my regional managers, and the Lululemon communications team. Within the week the post was removed and a statement from Lululemon read, "This is not a Lululemon forum and it does not represent the company's views."

My phone was lit up by calls from local, national, and global media. My name and face were showing up on my Google alerts left and right. One of my best friends I grew up with in Tacoma reached out to say, "I just saw you on television." I started to lose sight of my purpose and where my energy was being placed. My upcoming workshop had been threatened by trolls to be infiltrated, I was berated online across the world, and I was terrified to leave my house. My digital sweatlife sessions were canceled with less than two weeks' notice. A global brand once ready to parade me across global digital networks to value my work and contribution oh so quickly recoiled from me as a hot flame. I requested internal conversations with the team on why I was not supported by the brand. Why didn't I get a say in the communications response? What role did I get to have in how my work was upheld? Instead, the internet took hold of the tag line "resist capitalism" paired with the analysis that Lululemon thrives because of capitalism and its billion-dollar revenue. The pressure from the public placed me in the crossfire, and I lost my foundation.

When I signed with this brand, I was signing up for their solidarity. In place, I received fickle allyship only when it benefitted their name and position for the good of diversity and inclusion work. This is the epitome of check-box allyship. Lululemon was willing to bring me on as an ambassador but wasn't willing to do the work it takes to bring trust from my community.

The upcoming months were incredibly challenging, sifting through the distraction of global news and worried phone calls. I'm grateful for my team who held me, my partner who wiped away my tears, and a community of people who, to this day, still have my back and co-conspire with me.

Release the Need to Conform

Through these experiences, I sat back and considered why I still had an internal need to fit in and please everyone. It brought me back to the comments on my report cards that said "Rebby would do much better if they applied themself" or "Rebby needs to focus more on classwork and be less distracted by their classmates." It brought me reflections on how long it took for me to come out, which I hid away in relationships that didn't always honor who I am. So naturally, I found the same behaviors show up in my working relationships and organizing.

White supremacy wants me tired and exhausted while still driving forward for production. Today, I push up against the need to exhaust myself to prove how hard I am working. Prioritizing rest is one of the most important practices in my life right now, particularly following the passing of my father in December 2020. I learned that I wasn't making space for my grief, and it bubbled up through emotional lash-outs and hiding away from my friends and community. It took diving in and saying out loud, "I am not okay," to be the one to receive healing, rather than give healing. I stepped back from teaching twelve to fifteen yoga classes a week on top of part-time and contract work.

The reality is that I have been raised with deep alignment to perfectionism, which fuels my conformity. I fitted myself into the picture others wanted me to be. I prioritized the benefits of alignment to larger systems, like global wellness brands and nonprofits, to build my foundation rather than remain at the margins of my community, working toward collective power. I lost sight of this fighting so hard to be the favorite child of a brand that may not have had space for me in the first place, at yoga studios who promised "inclusion" but placed the emotional labor on my heart to guide them through the process, and even in friendships and relationships where my wholeness was not valued.

The expectations placed on me in my schooling and early career created an internal dialogue that compared me to my peers, strived for perfection, and overworked for very little compensation or appreciation. This spilled over into myself and my own expression. I fought to meet the stereotypes as a thin, muscular, feminine yoga instructor, dressed head to toe in the most expensive yoga pants, forming my body into challenging advanced shapes. I made this to mean that I was a successful yoga instructor and attempted to build a following from that persona. The reality was that I felt scared to live authentically, afraid that I would be outcast or turned away, as I had been in college.

Through these steps on my journey, I had to get clear with myself and what it looks like to be in solidarity with myself. To turn my attention inward to see myself in the mirror and love every bit of me. To release the headlines from elected officials who introduce legislation to limit my existence in this world. I began to release the need to educate communities who aren't willing to do the work. To heal my burnout with rest and rejuvenation and undoing the harms I've faced while laying myself on the line for the learning of others.

My liberation today looks like centering myself and my healing journey. It looks like a stronger capacity to say no to engagements that create a fishbowl for my trauma, placing me in the center of harm for the learning of those in the room. It only took me thirty-three years to get here, and I am glad to have made it. Now I am able to take these learnings and hold space for my community to also be in their choice and find time to be seen, which can lead to the collective liberation we seek.

While life during the first year of the pandemic was isolating, it simultaneously brought me closer to transgender and nonbinary yoga teachers from across the US on Zoom. We created a virtual space to exist and share our raw thoughts about the challenges we were facing with employment, grief, and fear. During our sessions I found community among the not-so-long-ago strangers. A few of us came together to offer a public workshop for yoga teachers and studio communities to learn about ways to support transgender and nonbinary people in yoga and wellness spaces. This was the foundation of my co-founding the Trans Yoga Project* alongside seven inspirational friends and now co-conspirators.

The Trans Yoga Project is a collaborative effort supporting the spiritual wellness of trans people through community (re)education, advocacy within the yoga and wellness industries, community building, and the creation of supportive and affirming content and guided practices by and for trans and

---

* Trans Yoga Project, https://transyogaproject.com/.

nonbinary people. We commit to internal and external work in service to ALL trans, nonbinary, and queer siblings, and thus we are vested in dismantling all systems of oppression, including white supremacy and capitalism, in all their manifestations.

This became the healing I needed. I had been spending the last few years pouring my energy into white cisgender people in yoga who weren't engaged in liberatory practices, who were content with the bare minimum of posting a black square on social media. Yet, along the way, I wasn't feeding my soul. I became tired and uninspired. I was hurting from lighting myself on fire to keep others warm.

Remain in the Work

In order to reach the liberation we seek, it is necessary to recognize the role to play in this work. To name when it is time to rest and heal, and when it is time to use your power to hold the door open for others to elevate.

My hope is that yoga studios, specifically those owned and run by white straight cisgender people, take active work to end tokenization and exploitation. Having studios run and led by white folks, while proudly selling local goods from BIPOC and LGBTQ creators and businesses, can be problematic when there is not a representation of BIPOC and LGBTQ people in studio leadership. This is a clear example of optical and performative allyship. When BIPOC and LGBTQ people are in decision-making positions within systems, it helps redistribute power and ensure that our voices are centered. Decisions about us should not be made without us.

Apparel lines have work to do by centering larger bodies and those with disabilities. List your sizes starting with your largest size: 6X–XS—and carry enough inventory for all sizes, rather than average sizes. Remove gender from clothing to center trans and gender queer people by listing clothing styles rather than gender expectations: fitted or relaxed fits. Carry apparel created by BIPOC and LGBTQ people, and release clothing that reinforces toxic positivity like "spiritual gangster" or "good vibes only."

For the white-led yoga festivals and community events, the work needed is for white folks to take a seat. The most common question I get asked by white cisgender women in yoga is, "How do I create a studio/class/festival that's inclusive for BIPOC LGBTQ people?" The only answer I have is: you don't. It's not your work to do. Your work is to redistribute the wealth and resources needed for BIPOC and LGBTQ people to lean into what is most needed for the community. Festivals led by white folks, bringing in presenters with identities often exploited by "Diversity and Inclusion (DEI)" work, will nearly always cause harm to those presenters. This is not an environment of equity, nor is it practicing co-conspiracy.

There are many costs in the work of solidarity. The cost of ignoring systemic harm by spiritually bypassing racism, transphobia, and ableism through performative allyship and toxic positivity. There is a cost to the ongoing centering of whiteness and alignment to dominant culture, particularly in a time when all communities are under attack by state and federal legislation seeking to limit and ban access to basic services like healthcare and an inclusive education.

For trans, queer, and people of color, now is the time to rest and heal. The weight of the attacks on our community is heavy, and it is not designed to be carried alone. We are the ones who keep us safe. May we continue to create the spaces we need and trust in community care.

This is all needed in the work of solidarity to actively dismantle the systems that impact yoga, wellness, fitness, and society at large. Taking care of our health and bodies is necessary work, and we deserve to do so with ease and calm. Let's work together to get there and continue the work to remain there.

Epilogue

JUSTICE ROE WILLIAMS

The fitness industry is not separate from any other industry in this economy. It is a part of a larger industrial complex, which advances a profit-driven relationship that influences and maintains our current social order. By defining the fitness-industrial complex—a system that is deeply invested in controlling how we see, move, and live in our bodies—we can better understand how expansive this network is. Examining this system helps us let go of the pervasive myth taught by the fitness industry: the idea of "perfection" and that our bodies are wrong, inferior, and need to be fixed. Most of all, this work uncovers our relationship with the industry and how we both conform to and are oppressed by these harmful ideas of perfection. The fitness industry is a part of our broken system, and it needs to be deconstructed and reframed to make space and create access for all our bodies. Just as activists have been working to deconstruct the military-industrial complex and the prison-industrial complex, the fitness-industrial complex is due for deep examination and critical reassessment.

This book is a call to action for trainers, coaches, and gym owners within the industry to move away from upholding the toxic ideology of physical "perfection" and to become a shield for our clients instead. In order to do this, we must identify the racist, sexist, classist, and ableist roots of eugenics within the beliefs and ideas that frame our industry. One example is our use of the body mass index (BMI), a formula created in the 1830s by Belgian astronomer, mathematician, statistician, and sociologist Lambert Adolphe

Jacques Quetelet.[1] For the unfamiliar, the formula for BMI uses weight and height to calculate this measure of "body mass" ($BMI=kg/m^2$), which is then evaluated against a chart that uses the factors of gender and age to determine if an individual is underweight, a healthy weight, overweight, or obese based upon their body mass index.

In creating this formula to calculate BMI, Quetelet relied on the idea of the "average man," which for him was a white, European man. This formula has since been inappropriately applied to swathes of populations who were not considered in its creation. Even more, this dynamic is the fundamental issue of so many measures used in fitness (and, one could argue, the existence of measures in the first place): the construction of the average body (as well as the ideally "healthy" body that is extrapolated from it) that is applied to everyone without consideration for the wide array of life experiences and embodiments that exist.

Healthcare providers, scientists, researchers, policymakers, and authors have used BMI to reinforce social biases against "larger" bodies in the name of promoting "health" and "wellness." Fitness professionals also reinforce these stigmas and disregard the person in front of them, seeing them as a project—something to be fixed rather than a person with their own goals, interests, and desires. Fitness professionals will also use BMI to make inappropriate assumptions about what people can do in terms of movement, regardless of an individual's demonstrated abilities of strength, flexibility, or cardiovascular capacity.

Science, and the authority it holds, has been used to reinforce our own personal ideas and standards around bodies, abilities, and beauty. This is the basis of eugenics. While dismissed as "unscientific" now, eugenics historically had, and continues to have, a hold on members of scientific and medical communities where science is used to reinforce racism, sexism, cisheteronormativity, ableism, nationalism, and more.

As coaches, we have to be accountable to the ideas that we validate and acknowledge the power we hold. When we conform to particular ideas, even when backed by science, and do not question the knowledge we possess and apply in our practices, we sustain our own subconscious desire to feel valued as an authority figure. We must acknowledge the power of the status quo and our complicity in upholding it, especially if we are naming ourselves as agents of change. Especially in the position of being a gatekeeper, where people are coming to us for information and insight about their body and movement, if we can't discuss the ways we hold power, then we cannot truly eradicate the ways we are oppressed or dismantle the systems of oppression we participate in.

Coaches have been taught that fitness and movement must be attached to a goal, event, or body aesthetic standard we are trying to reach. Understanding the business of fitness will help us understand why we are taught that our role as coaches and trainers is to fix the body. We are selling the lies that fitness will correct our bodies, heal our illness, and ensure longevity. Throughout this book you have heard from coaches, trainers, and athletes about their personal experiences within the industry. Through exposing ourselves to these shared experiences, we find respectful ways to be in space with each other. Exposure is key to understanding and adapting to the space and community around us.

Exposure is the most important part of unlearning. During our course "Deconstructing the Fitness Industrial Complex," we share video footage of two major events with our participants to consider and reflect upon. The first is of the police's reaction to protesters of George Floyd's murder on May 25, 2020. In it, we see the raging attacks against protesters of all body shapes, size, gender, ability, age, and race—basically anyone who spoke up against the police brutality that led to Floyd's death. Even though George Floyd's death sparked a national outcry for racial justice, it was just one of many deaths within the Black community at the hands of police brutality and white supremacy in 2020.

Immediately after watching that video, we share a video of the insurrection at the Capitol on January 6, 2021, that happened after former President Trump lost the 2020 presidential election to President Joe Biden. Again, we see violence, but from the protesters against the cops. I remember seeing angry white people, mainly men, make their way into the Capitol building with the intention to murder the lawmakers inside, and they met little resistance. We watch as cops are stunned, as they step aside letting the pro-testers do as they pleased. We then ask our participants, "Whose bodies are deemed valuable?" They answer: white male bodies are most valued.

By using this as our introduction to the course, the participants see how white men have more authority, access to power and resources, and bodies that are deemed more valuable in our society. The overturning of Roe v. Wade on June 24, 2022, denying people the right to an abortion, is a painful reminder of the authority that white cisgender men have over our bodies. This is also true within the fitness industry, which operates and is influenced by the very same ideals, giving white men the authority to define and dictate what fitness and wellness mean. The white male per-spective is reinforced by the industry—from the curriculum for our college courses and fitness certifications (and who that's created for) to who the larger industry highlights as our leaders.

It's Not Our Bodies That Need to Be Fixed!

Deconstructing fitness means understanding how fitness acts within a larger web of industries and interlocking systems of power. It is examining how fitness is used as a tool to mold us into labor and productivity-driven commodities and consumers. It is interrogating how fitness reinforces white beauty standards and values. One of the first steps to demystify and detach movement from the fitness-industrial complex is by meeting bodies—our clients' bodies and our own—where they are at.

"Meeting bodies where they are at" is a social justice framework. It means understanding that we must question the ideas and standards that we hold about bodies and their abilities and how we unintentionally use these stan-dards to validate this need to "fix" bodies. This framework allows us the space to value and honor all bodies and abilities in their natural state, with the understanding that all bodies—and movement in those bodies—are ever-changing and unique.

Meeting bodies where they are at helps coaches apply a social justice lens to their work with clients. This is the process of unlearning toxic ideas that we have internalized from certifying organizations and institutions. While deconstructing the ideas that we have learned about athleticism and ability that are ingrained within the fitness industry, we are using ourselves, our bodies, to reframe what movement looks like.

Those of us within the industry have to understand that we don't define what fitness is to our clients. The fitness-industrial complex says that fitness only happens in certain spaces, according to certain rules, and is only achievable by certain types of bodies. We have to unlearn this schema and emphasize justice in our discussions with clients. We need to help everyone see how we embody fitness beyond the ideals and understanding we were taught.

Do All Bodies Need to Push, Pull, Hinge, and Squat?

When we are thinking about fitness and our unique body's relationship to movement, are we taking into consideration the true needs of our clients? This is connected to the ways that we assess our clients. We learn that our bodies need to be able to do specific movements that we've deemed productive or necessary, therefore creating the standards that we all follow to guide us in our relationships with movement and our bodies. Deconstructing fitness means centering the needs of the individual, not an abstract standard of what they should be.

Part of the work of coaches and trainers is letting go of ego. When my mentor told me that we learn more from bodies than books, it confirmed what I had been feeling: that as a coach I am learning more from my clients than what I learned in order to pass my certification. It is not my job to try to "fix" someone's body, and it's important for me to know the difference between assisting a movement pattern and fixing something. We acknowledge that bodies are different and that basic movements will look different in different bodies, but applied science erases that diversity and says that all of these movements should look the same. If we move with the understanding that bodies don't need fixing, we can let go of making bodies meet someone else's expectations and just allow physical movement to happen.

Bringing in More Bodies: Inclusion beyond Accommodations

Today and every day, it is the work of fitness professionals to create spaces where we can think critically about our practices and approaches to movement and our own and others' fitness journeys. We have to step away from tools and assessments that inform us there is something wrong with our bodies. Otherwise, we risk othering any embodiment besides able-bodied, cisgender, white, heterosexual men—the body that serves as the standard for these assessments and demands alignment of other bodies toward it. It is not our place to be in the business of oppressing others, which is why we say that inclusion also goes beyond accommodations.

Accommodations—while necessary and something that everyone deserves in their daily life including and beyond fitness spaces—are not what inherently creates belonging. If the space you're working in or the practices you're using are still holding embodiments of dominant culture at its center and as a goal to achieve, then you are only making someone more included in their own oppression. What creates belonging in a radical, authentic sense is digging up the roots of the systems we engage in. It is recognizing these truths about the fitness-industrial complex, confronting them, recognizing our complicity in them, and figuring out how to begin building new practices through real relationships that support individuals in their own bodies, not just the one that traditional fitness envisions they should strive toward. This is what we mean when we say that fitness should be a way to celebrate and honor our bodies. Our role should always be collaborating with clients and asking questions in order to create experiences to meet our clients where they are at in their bodies.

An important part of this process is the language we use. For example, this means recognizing how sentiments like "no pain, no gain" don't help us understand those in our community who experience chronic pain. It means reflecting on the role of militarization within the fitness industry[2] to consider the way we give cues, the way we choose to encourage people, and the standards we hold them to that might be preventing us from creating ways to communicate and meet our clients just as they are. Erasing the standards we hold around strength, power, and ability allows us to change our viewpoint and approach and creates better spaces where more of our community feel invested, seen, and able to move.

Throughout this book, you have received a broad perspective of both experiences within the fitness-industrial complex and some concrete ways to reframe what movement means for all bodies. You have heard some conventional and unconventional coaching ideas and practices. You have also heard from coaches and athletes of all body shapes, sizes, and identities who have successfully shifted the narrative for their bodies and also their clients' relationship to movement. This book is a part of an overarching conversation we need to be a part of, especially when talking about how our bodies experience movement. A conversation means that there will be disagreement and different perspectives; the various chapters of the book highlight some different perspectives. This book also shows us that there is not just one way to move and be in our bodies.

So why do we focus on inclusion, and what does it have to do with fitness? My hope is to share some language that helps us understand how these oppressive ideas separate us from our own bodies and cause us to hate the erasure of our bodies in relation to the world. We have to see that societal falsehoods ("isms") have ripped us apart at the seams. Inclusion can't be about just one experience but must involve exposing ourselves to many different experiences. We must constantly acknowledge that we are a larger community working together to eradicate these toxic ideas that we have learned about our bodies. Today and every day, it is the work of Fitness 4 All Bodies to create spaces where we can think critically about our practice as fitness professionals. Every day we take another step in deconstructing the fitness-industrial complex together.

About the Editors

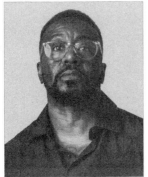

Justice Roe Williams (he/him, Boston, MA) is a certified personal trainer, head coach at Kettlebell Justice, founder of the Queer Gym Pop Up and Body Image 4 Justice, and executive director of Fitness 4 All Bodies.

Based in Boston, Williams is a trans, body-positive activist who has been creating safe spaces for queer and trans bodies since 2013. He advocates for fitness being for everyone and the importance of trainers and fitness professionals using their status as gatekeepers to "act as a shield" to protect their clients and create safe, affirming practices and spaces.

A key component of his work has been working with people of all backgrounds to address and dismantle toxic masculinity and how it operates within white supremacist patriarchal culture—particularly in fitness. His work has been featured in Refinery29, *Good Housekeeping*, NPR, Pink News, Boston Neighborhood Network News, and more.

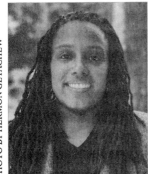

Roc Rochon (they/them, Tallahassee, FL) is a cultural worker and founder of Rooted Resistance, a space committed to reimagining bodywork for queer, transgender, and nonbinary people in the US South. Roc is currently a doctoral candidate in the Department of Sport Management at Florida State University (traditional and ancestral territory of the Apalachee Nation, the Muscogee Creek Nation, the Miccosukee Tribe of Florida, and the Seminole Tribe of Florida) with a focus on sociocultural aspects of sport and physical culture.

Roc's studies are concerned with unsettling "sport" as a politicized cultural form through understanding how histories of land, power, subjugation, and colonialism interact with bodies (human and nonhuman). Most importantly, Roc's interest is in narrative stories and the ways that Black queer, trans, and nonbinary folk create bodywork counterspaces that tend to collective Black life.

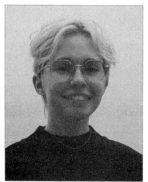

PHOTO BY NIKHITA NALLA

Lawrence Koval (they/he, Chicago, IL) received their folklore MA from UNC Chapel Hill in 2021. Their thesis work, "Explorations in the Inclusive Fitness Movement: Community Voices & Visions," was inspired by both their experience working in the fitness industry and the incredible activists, professionals, and collectives focused on imagining gyms and studios as spaces to engage in alternate, visionary economies of care.

Having worked in the fitness and wellness industry since 2011 as a yoga, cycle, and group fitness instructor, and going on to obtain their personal training certification in 2021, Lawrence finds it imperative that people consider the way politics are enacted and produced in fitness spaces. Their work continues to explore sports and physical culture especially related to media through the lens of queer studies, critical disability studies, and cultural studies.

About the Contributors

Beck M. Beverage (Portland, OR) — In their early twenties, Beverage developed a passion for functional fitness. They became a personal trainer, corrective exercise specialist, and even owned a fitness studio, Sweet Momentum Fitness, in Portland. Beverage was (and still is) passionate about working with people who don't usually feel comfortable in traditional gyms and fitness spaces. As they were learning and working with more people, Beverage started noticing some things in their body, and in the experiences of the people they were working with. How challenging it is to "feel" certain exercises, how hard it can be for folks to find themselves in space, and the way fear, anxiety, stress, trauma, and depression impact movement.

Beverage dove into studying all things neurobiology, fitness, somatics, philosophy, sociology, history, and more. They've spent the last seven-plus years developing a unique approach that blends the best information from a variety of disciplines.

Beverage is proudly transgender, intersex, queer, and neurodivergent. Their number one goal is to hold space for people of all bodies, backgrounds, and ability levels. You are welcome here.

Beverage believes that it's important to know the bodies we have, as opposed to a trying to achieve a body that is different from our own. They do not promote or engage with weight-loss or other aesthetic goals (muscle building, getting toned, etc.).

John R. Bridger (Fort Collins, CO) — John Bridger is a licensed clinical-community psychologist who has a private practice in Fort Collins, Colorado. John specializes in building authentic relationships to collaboratively develop resilience and healing with those navigating the complex impacts of acute, interpersonal, intergenerational, and collective trauma.

M Camellia (Washington, DC) — Melanie Camellia (née Williams), E-RYT 200 & YACEP, is a fat, queer, nonbinary yoga teacher and accessibility advocate in Washington, DC, called to create profoundly inclusive spaces for self-inquiry and the inward journey by integrating spiritual teachings and accessible, trauma-informed movement practices with the spirit of social justice. Melanie believes that the goal of yoga, as of life, is collective liberation, and in turn challenges contemporary yoga practitioners to dismantle the oppressive systems and beliefs, within themselves and society at large, that hold us all back.

Melanie's classes often include functional movement practices alongside more traditional alignment-based postures and flow elements that link breath and body. In addition to teaching group and private yoga classes, Melanie offers workshops that explore queer identity, body image, desire, pleasure, and agency. They champion diversity and equity in the yoga industry as a member of the Yoga & Body Image Coalition leadership team. They continue to serve as an expert adviser on diversity, accessibility, and ethics for the Yoga Alliance Standards Review Project and currently work with Accessible Yoga to help bring their teacher trainings and conferences to an ever-growing list of cities internationally.

Dr. Marcia Dernie (South Florida) — Marcia is a Haitian American, physical therapist, Black creative, spoonie, and powerlifting strongwoman living in South Florida (on Seminole Land). Marcia was always an athletic person but didn't begin her lifting journey until 2010. After her first powerlifting competition in 2011, she competed several times a year at national level meets and held state records. By 2016 Marcia found herself with a body that no longer listened or performed as expected.

After two years of inconsistent performances, Marcia shifted her focus to the equally demanding but more flexible sport of Strongman. In her first year of competing, she qualified for 2019 nationals in two different federations. Nursing an undiagnosed condition takes a great amount of soul searching and mental fortitude to stay focused and adapt accordingly in a world built for the able-bodied.

Marcia is the owner of Move with Marcia, an online resource and You-Tube channel for physical therapy and yoga.

Damali Fraiser (Brampton, ON) — Born from a story of healing and reflection, Lift Off Strength & Wellness is led by Damali Fraiser, an SFG Level 2 certified kettlebell instructor and Poo Choi Kru. She began her kettlebell journey from her passion for Muay Thai.

Muay Thai is referred to as the "Art of Eight Limbs" as it makes use of punches, kicks, elbows, and knee strikes. You might be wondering how that relates? Every fighter requires an effective strength and conditioning program that is efficient and creates density, not bulk. Functional training is about getting stronger at compound movements you can use in real life to be more efficient and prevent injuries. Implementing a kettlebell practice as a functional training tool toward greater strength opens a world of opportunity for everyone.

Asher Freeman (Philadelphia, PA) — Owner and founder of Nonnormative Body Club, Freeman is a Philadelphia-based nonbinary and trans personal trainer dedicated to smashing fatphobic, cisnormative, misogynist, ableist, and racist myths about our health and bodies. They have been featured in the *New York Times* and in *Self* magazine with several other trainers listed on the Body Positive Fitness Finder.

Sonja R. Price Herbert (Atlanta, Georgia) — Sonja is an antiracism educator/consultant for Pilates/fitness, activist, Pilates instructor, social worker, writer, and founder/creator of Black Girl Pilates, which is a platform highlighting and supporting Black women-identifying Pilates instructors globally. Sonja is committed to Black representation within fitness and improving the health and wellness in the Black community through writing, speaking, and advocacy.

Adele Jackson-Gibson (Oakland, CA) — Adele Jackson-Gibson is a certified fitness coach, model, and writer based in Oakland. She earned her master's in journalism from NYU, her bachelor's in literature from Yale University, and has since written for various sports, fitness, beauty, and culture outlets.

Rebby Kern (Charlotte, NC) — Rebby is the education policy director at Equality NC and has worked in LGBTQ activism over the past decade. Rebby works full-time as a social justice warrior supporting LGBTQ youth across the state and region through education policy, youth programming, anti-racism work, and leadership development.

After completing their yoga teacher training in 2018, Rebby has been teaching yoga in studios, yoga for queer youth, yoga with horses, Head Start programming to introduce yoga to children, and yoga in many spaces in the city of Charlotte. As a Lululemon Ambassador, Rebby is able to lead in power in the Charlotte community and beyond. Rebby is the first nonbinary person of color to represent Lululemon in the region and continues to uplift voices of LGBTQ and BIPOC people who often don't find themselves represented within the Lululemon brand.

Opportunities to lead social justice work within yoga spaces presented themselves, and Rebby began working with Jasmine Hines and Amplify & Activate to teach yoga as a tool for self-care and social justice. This work stems from antiracism work and challenges current practices and ethics present in yoga studios and fitness spaces. From that work stemmed Rebby's Race, Gender & Bias workshops, facilitated for YTTs, studio staff, and virtual workshops during COVID-19.

In 2020 Rebby joined forces with SweatNET Charlotte to localize their work within yoga and fitness spaces and create a more equitable, accessible sweat experience for each person who seeks it. Rebby also completed Yoga 12-Step Recovery Training, returning to the foundation of their own practice to explore an addiction recovery model that connects yoga, neuroscience, and the practical tools of 12-step programs.

Kanoelani Patterson (Lawton, OK) — Kanoelani Patterson is thirty-nine years old and a SHW fat-positive powerlifter. They currently hold a master's degree in social work (MSW). Social work, social justice, and marginalized communities have their heart. Patterson currently is working on licensure in social work, and their focus is working with children and teens. They practice an antidiet philosophy and believe you can be active without striving for intentional weight loss. They eat intuitively and believe that food is more than calories and fuel: food is culture, food is love, food is memories, and more. Patterson believes that freedom can be found in movement and food, but to do that we have to decolonize the way we view the two. **we are enough as we are** and should be affirmed as such.

Sunaina Rangnekar (Denver, Colorado) — Sunaina is a multidimensional infinite energy, captured within their body bag. They identify as a nonbinary yoga visionary, mentor, and cultural artivist. Currently, they reside on the unseeded ancestral homelands of the Apache, Ute, Cheyenne, and Arapahoe Nations colonized as Denver, Colorado. It is their aspiration to create a global, community-centered world that focuses on individual and collective healing through living in one's own unique truth. They are currently partnered with Alchemystic Studio, an inclusive, queer, Indian-run yoga studio that alchemizes the heart of an activist with the mind of a yogi. Currently, they mentor alongside Susanna Barkataki on her 300 Hour Embrace Yoga's Roots teacher training. They hold spaces to reclaim yoga, decolonize minds, and abolish oppressive systems that affect us at an energetic and societal level. Through their embodied yoga practice, Sunaina brings a new and unique lens to the yogic path.

Notes

Introduction

1 Patti DeRosa and Ulric Johnson, "The 10 Cs: A Model of Diversity Awareness and Social Change," in ChangeWorks Consulting, Transformation for a Better Future, 2002, 1–8.

2 Chris Lovett, "Health, Wellness Event at Fitness Center," interview video, Boston Neighborhood News, 2013, https://vimeo.com/77415779.

3 Quincy Walters, "'Queer Gym' Empowers LGBTQ+ Clients, Both Physically and Mentally," NPR, October 15, 2019, www.npr.org/2019/10/15/769023643/queer-gym-empowers-lgbtq-clients-both-physically-and-mentally.

4 "The Health of Lesbian, Gay, Bisexual and Transgender (LGBT) Persons in Massachusetts," a survey of health issues comparing LGBT persons with their heterosexual and non-transgender counterparts, Massachusetts Department of Public Health, July 2009, 1–24, www.mass.gov/files/documents/2016/07/ra/lgbt-health-report.pdf.

5 Eve Tuck and K. Wayne Yang, "Decolonization Is Not a Metaphor," *Decolonization: Indigeneity, Education & Society* 1, no. 1 (September 8, 2012).

6 David L. Andrews, "Kinesiology's Inconvenient Truth and the Physical Cultural Studies Imperative," *Quest* 60, no. 1 (2008): 45–62.

Chapter 1

1 Samantha Riedel, "Remembering Rita Hester, Who Changed What It Means to Remember Trans Lives," them, March 31, 2022, www.them.us/story/rita-hester-trans-remembrance-visibility-memorial.

2 Ilya Parker, "What Is Toxic Fitness Culture?" Decolonizing Fitness, June 17, 2020, https://decolonizingfitness.com/blogs/decolonizing-fitness/what-is-toxic-fitness-culture.

3 Audre Lorde, "There Is No Hierarchy of Oppressions," in "Homophobia and Education," special issue, *Interracial Books for Children Bulletin* 14, no. 3-4 (1983): 9, http://digital.library.wisc.edu/1711.dl/Literature.CIBCBulletinv14n0304.

4 Carol Hanisch, "The Personal Is Political," accessed July 17, 2022, http://www .carolhanisch.org/CHwritings/PIP.html.

Chapter 2

1 David S. Churchill, "Making Broad Shoulders: Body-Building and Physical Culture in Chicago 1890–1920," *History of Education Quarterly* 48, no. 3 (2008): 341–70, www.jstor.org/stable/20462241.

2 Churchill, "Making Broad Shoulders," 347.

3 Siobhan Somerville, "Scientific Racism and the Emergence of the Homosexual Body," *Journal of the History of Sexuality* 5, no. 2 (1994): 243–66, www.jstor.org /stable/3704199.

4 Somerville, "Scientific Racism," 256.

5 Somerville, 257.

6 Somerville, 250.

7 Churchill, "Making Broad Shoulders," 350.

8 Churchill.

9 Churchill, 344.

10 "YMCA History: The Founding Years," YMCA, accessed September 20, 2022, www.ymca.org/who-we-are/our-history/founding-years.

11 Churchill, "Making Broad Shoulders," 353.

12 Churchill, 353.

13 Churchill, 354.

14 Chris Wienke, "Negotiating the Male Body: Men, Masculinity, and Cultural Ideals," *Journal of Men's Studies* 6, no. 3 (June 1998): 255–82, https://doi .org/10.1177/106082659800600301.

15 Natalia Petrzela, "Thanks, Gender! An Intellectual History of the Gym," in *American Labyrinth: Intellectual History for Complicated Times*, ed. Raymond Haberski, Jr., and Andrew Hartman (Ithaca, NY: Cornell University Press, 2018), 86–103.

16 Alan Klein, *Little Big Men: Bodybuilding Subculture and Gender Construction* (Albany, NY: SUNY Press, 1993).

17 Petrzela, "Thanks, Gender!" 93.

18 Petrzela, 93.

19 Petrzela.

20 Petrzela.

21 Klein, *Little Big Men*.

22 Petrzela, "Thanks, Gender!"

23 Klein, *Little Big Men*, 162.

24 Wienke, "Negotiating the Male Body"; Klein, *Little Big Men*.

25 Shelly A. McGrath and Ruth A. Chananie-Hill, "Big Freaky-Looking Women": Normalizing Gender Transgression through Bodybuilding," *Sociology of Sport Journal* 26, no. 2 (2009): 235–54, https://doi.org/10.1123/ssj.26.2.235.

26 Petrzela, "Thanks, Gender!"

27 Klein, *Little Big Men*, 161.

28 Moya Bailey, "Misogynoir in Medical Media: On Caster Semenya and R. Kelly," *Catalyst: Feminism, Theory, Technoscience* 2, no. 2 (2016): 1–31, https://doi.org/10.28968/cftt.v2i2.28800.

29 Bailey, "Misogynoir in Medical Media," 10.

30 Bailey, 4.

31 Bailey, 11.

32 Maxine Leeds Craig and Rita Liberti, "'Cause That's What Girls Do': The Making of a Feminized Gym," *Gender and Society* 21, no. 5 (2007): 676–99, www.jstor.org/stable/27641005.

33 Stephanie E. Coen, Joyce Davidson, and Mark W. Rosenberg, "'Where Is the Space for Continuum?' Gyms and the Visceral "Stickiness" of Binary Gender," *Qualitative Research in Sport, Exercise, and Health* 13, no. 4 (2020), 537–53, https://doi.org/10.1080/2159676X.2020.1748897.

34 Coen, Davidson, and Rosenberg, 5.

35 Coen, Davidson, and Rosenberg.

36 Leeds Craig and Liberti, "'Cause That's What Girls Do."

37 Leeds Craig and Liberti.

38 Robyn Longhurst, "Queering Body Size and Shape: Performativity, the Closet, Shame and Orientation," in *Queering Fat Embodiment*, ed. Cat Pausé, Jackie Wykes, and Samantha Murray (Burlington, VT: Ashgate, 2014), 13–25; Caleb Luna, "The Gender Nonconformity of My Fatness," The Body Is Not an Apology, August 10, 2018, https://thebodyisnotanapology.com/magazine/the-gender-nonconformity-of-my-fatness/; Margitte Kristjansson, "Fashion's 'Forgotten Woman': How Fat Bodies Queer Fashion and Consumption," in *Queering Fat Embodiment*, ed. Cat Pausé, Jackie Wykes, and Samantha Murray (Burlington, VT: Ashgate, 2014), 131–46.

39 Cheryl Frazier and Nadia Medhi, "Forgetting Fatness: The Violent Co-optation of the Body Positivity Movement," *Debates in Aesthetics* 16, no. 1 (2021), http://debatesinaesthetics.org/debates-in-aesthetics-vol-16-no-1/#FRAZIERMEHDI.

40 Shari L. Dworkin and Faye Linda Wachs, *Body Panic: Gender, Health, and the Selling of Fitness* (New York: NYU Press, 2009).

41 Liat Ben-Moshe, *Decarcerating Disability: Deinstitutionalization and Prison Abolition* (Minneapolis: University of Minnesota Press, 2020).

42 Alexis Pauline Gumbs, "Freedom Seeds: Growing Abolition in Durham, North Carolina," in *Abolition Now! Ten Years of Strategy and Struggle against the Prison Industrial Complex*, ed. CR-10 Publications Collective (AK Press, 2008), 145.

Chapter 3

1 Heather Ashbach, "Where Does Fat Phobia Come From?" University of California News, August 15, 2019, www.universityofcalifornia.edu/news/fat-phobia.
2 Audre Lorde, "Uses of the Erotic: The Erotic as Power," originally delivered at the Fourth Berkshire Conference on the History of Women, Mount Holyoke College, August 25, 1978. Originally published as a pamphlet by Out & Out Books, distributed by Crossing Press.

Chapter 5

1 *Merriam-Webster*, s.v. "athletic," accessed September 20, 2022, www.merriam-webster.com/dictionary/athletic.
2 Amy Bass, "'Slave Genes' Myth Must Die," Salon, July 25, 2012, www.salon.com/2012/07/25/michael_johnsons_gold_medal_in_ignorance/.
3 Rebecca Scott, Julien Cayla, and Bernard Cova, "Selling Pain to the Saturated Self," *Journal of Consumer Research* 44, no. 1 (2017): 22–43, https://doi.org/10.1093/jcr/ucw071.
4 "What Is Rhabdo?," Centers for Disease Control and Prevention, April 22, 2019, www.cdc.gov/niosh/topics/rhabdo/what.html.
5 bell hooks, *All About Love: New Visions* (New York: Harper Perennial, 2001), 5.
6 Toni Morrison, *Jazz* (New York: Alfred A. Knopf, 1992), 228.
7 Mae Rice, "Here's Why You Unconsciously Copy Other People's Mannerisms," *Discovery*, August 1, 2019, www.discovery.com/science/copy-other-peoples-mannerisms.

Chapter 7

1 Pilates Foundation, "The History of Pilates," accessed September 20, 2022, www.pilatesfoundation.com/pilates/the-history-of-pilates/.
2 Joseph H. Pilates, *Pilates' Return to Life through Contrology*, 2nd ed. (Pilates Method Alliance, 2012).

Chapter 9

1 Peter Gray, *Free to Learn: Why Unleashing the Instinct to Play Will Make Our Children Happier, More Self-Reliant, and Better Students for Life* (New York: Basic Books, 2013).

Chapter 11

1 Margaret K. Bass, "On Being a Fat Black Girl in a Fat-Hating Culture," in *Recovering the Black Female Body: Self-Representation by African American Women*, ed. Michael Bennett and Vanessa Dickerson (New Brunswick, NJ: Rutgers, 2000), 219–30.

2 Theodore Isaac Rubin, *Alive and Fat and Thinning in America* (New York: Putnam, 1978).

3 Danielle M. Ely and Anne K. Driscoll, "Infant Mortality in the United States, 2020: Data From the Period Linked Birth/Infant Death File," *National Vital Statistic Report* 71, no. 5 (September 29, 2022): 3. https://www.cdc.gov/nchs/data/nvsr/nvsr71/nvsr71-05.pdf

4 Malcolm X, "Speech to Women" (speech, Los Angeles, California, May 22, 1962), Face 2 Face Africa, https://face2faceafrica.com/article/heres-the-full-malcolm-x-speech-about-black-women-displayed-by-megan-thee-stallion-on-snl.

Chapter 12

1 Katarina Wind, "Why I No Longer Prescribe Weight Loss, Calculate BMI, or Use the Term 'Obesity,'" University of British Columbia, Faculty of Medicine, May 3, 2022, https://thischangedmypractice.com/why-i-no-longer-prescribe-weight-loss.

2 A. E. Kasardo and M. C. McHugh, "From Fat Shaming to Size Acceptance: Challenging the Medical Management of Fat Women," in *The Wrong Prescription for Women: How Medicine and Media Create a Need for Treatments, Drugs, and Surgery*, ed. Maureen C. McHugh and Joan C. Chrisler (Santa Barbara, CA: Praeger, 2015), 179–201.

Chapter 13

1 Kenneth Jones and Tema Okun, "White Supremacy Culture," in *Dismantling Racism: A Resource Book for Social Change Groups* (ChangeWorks 2001).

2 Lama Rod Owens, *Love and Rage* (Berkeley, CA: North Atlantic Books, 2020).

3 Michelle Cassandra Johnson, *Skill in Action* (Portland, OR: Shambala, 2017), 72–75.

4 Chris Isidore, "Target's $20 Million Answer to Transgender Bathroom Boycott," CNNMoney, August 17, 2016, https://money.cnn.com/2016/08/17/news/companies/target-bathroom-transgender/index.html.

5 Jamila Thomas and Brianna Agyemang, hosts, *The Show Must Be Paused* (podcast), www.instagram.com/theshowmustbepaused.

6 Jessica Bursztynsky and Sarah Whitten, "Instagram Users Flood the App with Millions of Blackout Tuesday Posts," CNBC, June 2, 2020, www.cnbc.com/2020/06/02/instagram-users-flood-the-app-with-millions-of-blackout-tuesday-posts.html.

7 Simi Olurin, Jordan Fitzgerald, Jordan Jenkins, Soleil Singh, and Allison Cho, guests, "Full Disclosure: Activism Beyond the Performance" *Yale Daily News Podcast* (podcast), November 11, 2020, https://soundcloud.com/ydnpodcast/full-disclosure-activism-beyond-the-performance.

8 "Ally or Co-conspirator?: What It Means to Act #InSolidarity," Move to End Violence, September 7, 2016, https://movetoendviolence.org/blog/ally-co-conspirator-means-act-insolidarity/.

9 Robin DiAngelo, *White Fragility: Why It's So Hard for White People to Talk about Racism* (Boston: Beacon, 2018).

10 Bobbie Harro, "The Cycle of Socialization," in *Readings for Diversity and Social Justice*, ed. Maurianne Adams, Warren J. Blumenfeld, Heather W. Hackman, Madeline L. Peters, and Xímena Zuñiga (London: Routledge, 2000), 45–52.

11 Cynthia Erivo, "Stand Up," Back Lot Music, 2019.

12 Meg Sangimino, "Toxic Positivity Has Become Trendy," Medium, August 12, 2019, https://medium.com/the-ascent/toxic-positivity-has-become-trendy-116573f4707c.

13 Tai Salih, "White Privilege in Yoga Pants: Spiritual Bypassing," Medium, June 18, 2020, https://medium.com/@taisalih/white-privilege-in-yoga-pants-spiritual-bypassing-a33b83232fb9.

14 Arundhati Baitmangalkar, "How We Can Work Together to Avoid Cultural Appropriation in Yoga," Yoga International, https://yogainternational.com/article/view/how-we-can-work-together-to-avoid-cultural-appropriation-in-yoga.

15 Philip Deslippe, "Yoga Landed in the U.S. Way Earlier Than You'd Think—And Fitness Was Not the Point," History.com, June 20, 2019, www.history.com/news/yoga-vivekananda-america.

Epilogue

1 Giles Yeo, "BMI: We Know It's Flawed, so Why Do We Still Use It?" Science Focus, July 6, 2021, www.sciencefocus.com/comment/bmi-we-know-its-flawed-so-why-do-we-still-use-it/.

2 Chris Hendershot, "The Militarized Gym," E-International Relations, March 24, 2015, www.e-ir.info/2015/03/24/the-militarized-gym/; Kevin McSorely, "Doing Military Fitness: Physical Culture, Civilian Leisure, and Militarism," Portsmouth University Research Portal, accessed July 19, 2022. https://core.ac.uk/download/pdf/44340375.pdf.

Index

About North Atlantic Books

North Atlantic Books (NAB) is an independent, nonprofit publisher committed to a bold exploration of the relationships between mind, body, spirit, and nature. Founded in 1974, NAB aims to nurture a holistic view of the arts, sciences, humanities, and healing. To make a donation or to learn more about our books, authors, events, and newsletter, please visit www.northatlanticbooks.com.